Kate Carr is a journalist who has worked for the *Sunday Times*, the *Times*, the *Daily Telegraph*, the *Mail on Sunday*, *Good House-keeping* and the *BBC*. This is her first book. She lives in London and Shropshire with her partner and two children.

It's Not Like That, Actually

A memoir of surviving cancer – and beyond

KATE CARR

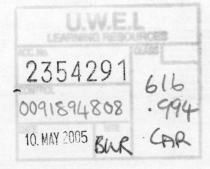
Vermilion
LONDON

1 3 5 7 9 10 8 6 4 2

First published in the United Kingdom in 2004 by
Vermilion, an imprint of Ebury Press
Random House UK Ltd
Random House
20 Vauxhall Bridge Road
London SW1V 2SA

Random House Australia (Pty) Ltd
20 Alfred Street, Milsons Point, Sydney,
New South Wales 2061, Australia

Random House New Zealand Limited
18 Poland Rd, Glenfield,
Auckland 10, New Zealand

Random House, South Africa (Pty) Limited
Endulini, 5a Jubilee Road, Parktown 2193, South Africa

Random House UK Limited Reg. No 954009
www.randomhouse.co.uk

Papers used by Vermilion are natural, recyclable products
made from wood grown in sustainable forests.

A CIP catalogue record for this book is available from the
British Library.

ISBN 0 09 189480 8

Typeset in Sabon by SX Composing DTP, Rayleigh, Essex

Printed and bound in Great Britain by
Mackays of Chatham plc, Chatham, Kent

To Simon, Lucian and Cosima, with love

Contents

ACKNOWLEDGEMENTS

With thanks to Sheila, Fred, Julie, Nellie, Sarah and Freddie Carr, Anna Barfield, Kerry Colletta, Dudley Sinnett, Charles Coombes, Adam Searle, Charles Lowdell, Anna Witham, Sally Parr, Gill Morgan, Felicity Rubinstein, Adam Phillips, Amanda Hemmings, Tim Lott, Sue Peart, Mick Brown, Emma Soames, Janette Marshall, Paula Reed, Joanna Bull, Lindsay Nicholson and Deirdre Vine. I wouldn't be here or have written this book without you.

AUTHOR NOTE

This book is about my experience of being diagnosed and treated for cancer, and what it is like to survive. It is not, however, a medical or reference book. All cancers are different and treatment protocols are constantly changing. They are also, I hope, improving. Anyone reading this book who is worried about their health should, in the first instance, contact their GP. Anyone who is in treatment, or post-treatment, for cancer and has concerns about their wellbeing should contact their oncologist. The only medical advice I feel I can give with any authority is that you should not ignore symptoms. At the back of the book is a list of organisations which may be helpful as a complement to medical care.

I did not die there, but I came close,
and there was a moment,
perhaps there were several moments,
when I tasted death, when I saw myself dead.
There is no cure for such an encounter.
Once it happens, it goes on happening;
you live with it for the rest of your life.

PAUL AUSTER, *THE LOCKED ROOM*

To do what you want is an everyday struggle.

MIUCCIA PRADA, *THE NEW YORKER*

Losing My Religion

By the time you read this book, I may be dead. Or dying. On the other hand, I may be just fine. The thing is, you see, I don't know for sure. You don't either, but unless you have been through what I have been through, you probably don't think about it much, perhaps not at all. I do, all the time, and what I'm thinking right now as I write this in the autumn of 2003 is that maybe there are some cancer cells in my body, cancer cells which escaped the surgery, chemotherapy and radiotherapy I had for breast cancer seven years ago when I was 39, swimming towards each other, eager to get together and form a tumour, a tumour that I won't know about until it has grown a bit and started getting bolshie, needing more room, more everything, making its presence, well, felt. If that happens, I'm in trouble, more trouble than I was first time round. You're always in trouble when cancer comes back. The doctors can try things but your chances are never as good second time round.

But maybe I am fine and will forever be fine. I simply don't know. The doctors don't know. There aren't any long-term statistics on the treatment I had and, anyway, cancer is predictable only in its unpredictability. The only way that I will ever get to say definitively that I had cancer and that, afterwards, I was fine is if I live another 20 years or so and find myself dying of something else. That's what surviving cancer is about. Waiting, wondering. Will my cancer come back or will I die of something else? It's also about knowing that however difficult that waiting and wondering is – and it is very difficult – there's no alternative. You have to get used to it, perhaps even persuade yourself that it's a great way to live. I have got used to it. I have worked hard to get used to it. I don't, however, think it's a great way to live. *To me, it is, as Homer Simpson says, crap on a crutch.*

I have never understood people who claim that their cancer is the best thing that has happened to them. What on earth were their lives like before? These triumph-over-tragedy types often write books, high as kites on their ability to get through their harrowing treatment, confessing their newfound appreciation of their wife, children, friends, cats, trees, whatever, and their determination to create a new and more meaningful life now that they have realised What Really Matters. I have some of these triumphal books on my shelves. The trouble is that the authors are, almost without exception, now dead. It's frustrating. I want to know how their more meaningful lives panned out, however briefly, because, in my experience, it is impossible to maintain that level of intensity about life for long, to make sweeping changes. Most people can't even change their hairstyle without a great deal of angst. However – and this is where things get complex, messy – I also know that it is impossible to go back to the old life after a cancer diagnosis. That familiar narrative arc, the crisis neatly resolved, doesn't seem to apply.

The story I tell myself about my life since I was diagnosed with cancer is forever changing and subject to change. I veer between thinking that I have merely lolloped along and that I have created something rather wonderful out of the ruins of my old life. What I never think is that the experience has been anything like I was led to expect, or like other people imagine it to be, which is why I have called this book *It's Not Like That, Actually*. It's what I have found myself repeatedly saying over the years. Maybe that's because the experience is poorly understood. Maybe it's just me. You decide.

In my opinion, I'm much like anyone else of my age and background. I was christened Kathryn, but started calling myself Kate when I was a teenager. I changed my name, or tinkered with it, because I was often called Kath which didn't feel like a name I could go far with. My father called me Kay, which I didn't mind, but I preferred Kate. It felt more me, something I could work with, and I often think the decision I made back then, over 30 years ago, says much about the way my mind works. Given a situation I don't like, I do something about it, maybe not much, but something. I'm not a drastic, melodramatic, revolutionary kind of person. I'm pragmatic, but I don't stay in one place. I look at what's there and I fiddle around with it until it's more to my liking.

I'm not sure where I got the name Kate from. Now I know a number of Kates. Then, I knew none. I was born in 1957 in east London and moved to Essex when I was one, first to Rainham and then to Romford where my peers were Christines and Janets and Janes and Catherines and Elizabeths and Deborahs,

3

and Kathryn was an anomaly. I liked the look of it, its angles and single descender, but I didn't like the sound of it, particularly when it got shortened to Kath. For one wild moment, I thought of changing it to October. I have no idea why. Some Seventies thing, I suppose. I probably flirted with Katy. On my bookshelf were the *What Katy Did* books by Susan Coolidge, those heart-warming stories about Katherine Carr, the doctor's daughter who fell off the swing and damaged her back but was so sweet and kind. But I probably dismissed it as twee. I wish I knew where Kate came from. It might tell me something about myself that I'd like to know.

But wherever it came from, it stuck. I've had nicknames, pet names. My sister Julie used to call me Miss Perfect. My sister Sarah, who was born when I was 11, called me Kark for a while. Simon, my partner for the past 27 years, calls me Hon, my friend Julia calls me Kato, and when I worked at the *Sunday Times* I was usually called Carr, except by my editor, Andrew Neil. Initially, he called me Kate, but when I became pregnant, he took to calling me Mother. I was – and possibly still am – also called other names behind my back. But Kate has been the fallback position.

In my twenties, when I was starting out as a journalist on women's magazines, I was asked by an exercise teacher I was interviewing if I had made up my name. It sounds like something out of *Compact*, she said. I barely remembered the soap set in a magazine office, but I knew what she meant. And I had and I hadn't made it up, and it did seem to have fictional legs. Susan Coolidge wasn't the only writer to have taken a fancy to it. A colleague at the *Sunday Times*, James, called a character in one of his novels Kate Carr. She was an overweight mother, so I wasn't thrilled. Harry, one of the literary editors, gallantly wrote a little piece saying how, in real life, I was rather elegant. Much later, Nick Hornby, in his novel *How to be Good*, called the proud doctor Katie Carr, which may or may not have been a coincidence. I had worked with him once and I had also, by then, stopped being a journalist and was working for Gilda's Club, a cancer support charity. Feeling paranoid, I wondered whether I, too, had become over-pleased with myself.

Kathryn has not disappeared completely though. In the past, various middle-aged male bosses have found it highly amusing for a friendly telling off. Miss Carr was another favourite in these circumstances. But nowadays the main offenders are people who know me from forms I have filled in. Doctors fall into this category.

I never really thought about this until I was told that I had cancer, mainly because I didn't go to my GP much, never developed much of a relationship with her and so never bothered to correct her. Then I started seeing doctors all the time, many different doctors, but over and over again. I got to know them a little. But I found myself letting them call me Kathryn. It turned out to be a form of self-protection, distancing. When they tell Kathryn this, that or the other, I can sometimes feel that they are not really talking to me, not the real me, and it makes it a little easier to hear what they are saying. Not much, but a little. The edge of formality which they unwittingly bring to the situation by calling me Kathryn allows me to respond formally, too, act a part, be grown-up, not scream, fall apart. It's useful. It keeps the emotion at bay briefly. And then I go home, Kate again, and absorb the information they have given me at my own pace. That's the theory anyway. But it's got a massive great hole in it because whenever they tell me something, it seems to change me. I'm never quite the same afterwards, never quite the same old Kate, so sometimes I wonder if I was right to believe that it was a name I could go far with.

It was important to me, you see, that going far, because I had come a long way and had every expectation of going further. I had made 'that journey', as my friend Lesley calls it. My parents gradually became more affluent as I was growing up. Not rich, but more affluent than their parents, despite having five children. As the eldest I had a bird's eye view of our changing fortunes. When I was 11, we moved to a bigger house in a nicer area. We always had a summer holiday, but by the time I had left home, the caravan holidays in Cornwall and Wales had been superseded by trips abroad.

And if my parents had been socially mobile, leaving behind their East End childhoods for the softer-edged suburbs, I was more so. They believed in education and, although they had both attended good schools, they had left young and completed their educations through evening classes, the Open University. I was one of four girls from my primary school to go to grammar school. I was the first person in my family to go to university. I was the first woman to become a managing editor at the *Sunday Times*, in charge of four sections of the paper, and only the second woman to edit the magazine. I was the only woman in the weekly conferences for a long time, and later, the only one with children. By the time I was 39, I was working at the *Mail on Sunday* and earning more money than I had ever dreamed of. I also had that long and happy relationship with Simon, who is not only funny and sexy, but uxorious in the nicest of ways. I had two incredible children, Lucian, six, and

Cosima, three, both beautiful, bright and charming. I had a flat in London, in a safe area, just off the Fulham Road, with a good state primary school nearby, and a cottage in Shropshire. Like everyone, I'd had some miserable times, struggles, but my considered take on life then was that I was happier than most, luckier than most. I believed that things could only get better way before Tony Blair, simply because that is what had always happened in my life. Well, it's sort of what I believed.

I say sort of because, like so many people who feel they have travelled far, like so many of my generation, I occasionally felt that this good fortune couldn't last, that something so quickly gained could as quickly be lost. I did not feel, as friends from wealthier backgrounds did, that I had a right to good fortune. But the anxiety was free-floating, not anchored to anything specific. I never, ever, thought that illness would queer the pitch for me. When I took out life insurance when Lucian was born, the broker suggested I take out dread disease insurance, too. Oh no, I said, quite confidently. *How wrong can a person be?*

So perhaps I was wrong about everything else, too. Maybe I need a more modern name, a modern name for modern times. Trinity perhaps, like the heroine of the Matrix films. But then again, does it really matter what I'm called? My life, my progress, has been pretty textbook and is, in so many ways, nothing to do with me, my determination and talents, and everything to do with the encouragement I was given, the economic climate and changing attitudes. And although I was shocked when I was told I had cancer, it was also a familiar enough story, a story of our time, almost a cliché: middle-class woman of 39 with two small children gets breast cancer, the dread disease of affluence.

The clichés ran out of steam after that though. The talk of the mother of all battles turned out to be nonsense. And the miracle of my survival? Look at you now, everyone says, frolicking in the sunshine with your golden children. You must wake up every morning full of joy, so glad to be alive. *I wish.* As I write this, I am a cancer survivor, a survivor of the disease, but also a survivor of cancer's clunky nomenclature, of the shedloads of absolute rubbish that is talked about the experience of cancer which has made my journey harder than it needed to be. This book is the story of what it was actually like for me to make that journey, the second great journey of my life, the so-called cancer journey, in a world in which Gloria Gaynor belting out 'I Will Survive' passes for a philosophy of survival.

2

Pressure Drop

The horrible stuff started in earnest at the beginning of June 1997. There had been a bit of a lead-up but not much. I can remember the room where it happened. It was a small room, painted white. There was a desk rammed against the wall. I sat to the left of the desk, facing the consultant. Behind him was the narrow bed on which I had just been examined. My back was up against the wall.

I was wearing a pale green silky twinset, a pair of agnès b black trousers and those French elastic pumps which were so popular back then. Jewellery? Pearls, a locket and Georg Jensen earrings. At my feet was my – one of my – Prada black nylon bag. My hair was long and thick, and layered. I was nervous, but only a little. I was sitting up straight.

None of these details is particularly important, but they are so vivid to me that it is as if there is a photograph of myself in that room that I have looked at many times. But I don't have a photograph. Who, after all, would take such a picture? But I can conjure up this visual memory, any time, anywhere, despite the fact that what I am remembering happened seven years ago. The image is burned into my brain. It is, to me, a picture of innocence, or more precisely, of the exact moment before I lost my innocence, the sense that I had some control over my life. A minute later, I was a different person. Not as different as I was to become – changed, gradually but inexorably, by the events that unfolded. But different enough.

If I tell you that I ended up binning those clothes and would have burned them if I could – tricky in a top-floor flat in the middle of London with no fireplace – despite the fact that they were almost new, it might give you some idea of how much I wish I could delete this picture from my memory bank. In the weeks following that consultation, every time I tried to wear those clothes I felt like a victim, as though I were about to walk in front of a firing squad. *And now, every time I gaze at that picture in my mind, I am overcome with despair.*

I rushed to that appointment with Mr Sinnett, the consultant at the Cromwell Hospital in west London. I've often wished I'd dawdled, been late, given myself a little more time in my old life. I was working on the *Mail on Sunday*'s *Night & Day* magazine at the time and the offices were round the corner in Kensington High Street, so it was only a matter of a 10-minute walk to the hospital. I'd taken the last appointment, at 7pm, because it was inconceivable to me at that time to make a doctor's appointment in work time, but I was still rushing because it's difficult to leave newspaper offices. There's always something going on. Sometimes it's urgent, sometimes it's not, but there are usually enough men around with wives at home to make the working day the wrong sort of flexitime. I didn't tell anyone where I was going. I was just another woman who had left early, probably something to do with her children. There were probably a few raised eyebrows.

I had, however, been to the hospital before, a couple of days before. I'd got this lump you see, in my right breast. I had discovered it a few weeks before when I was in Shropshire at the cottage. I don't know exactly when I discovered it. I didn't write it in my diary. The date is lurking in there somewhere between my sister Sarah's wedding and Simon and Lucian and Cosima's birthdays. What I do know is that, when I discovered it, I was in the bathroom which, like all the rooms, has views over fields and faraway hills. I was looking, staring really, out of the window which I often do. Our flat in London is on a noisy, busy road in what's sometimes called Chelsea, sometimes Earl's Court, the horizon, the sky chopped up, obscured by other houses and flats, so I like to lose myself in looking when I can. And suddenly I felt compelled to touch my breast. I don't know why, I just did, and I could feel something hard, a clearly defined lump or ridge, I wasn't sure which. But I only felt it for a second because my hand bounced off my body and I couldn't get it to touch my breast again. It was as if there was a force field round it. I turned to look in the mirror. I stared into my eyes. What are you thinking? I asked myself. This is what I was thinking.

This is going to take everything you've got.

There are two ways of looking at that thought. I was looking at both of them at the same time. Then I looked out of the window again. In the garden, I could see Simon with Lucian and Cosima. It was sunny. They were having fun. I felt as though I was looking down on them from a great height. They seemed very far away.

And yet, like my hand, I bounced back. I told Simon. He was concerned but not overly. It couldn't possibly be anything, he said. Don't be daft. You're only 39. Back in London, I made an appointment with my GP, but otherwise I carried on as normal. I went to work. Simon went to work. Lucian went to school, Cosima to nursery. They came home to Kerry, our nanny, part-babe, part-Mary Poppins, who we all adored and who had been part of our lives since Lucian was born. We went to Shropshire at weekends. *Same old, same old*.

This wasn't as difficult as it sounds. I found that I couldn't actually absorb the fact that I had a lump in my breast. I couldn't work out where it fitted in the story I told myself about my life and I had no desire to try and make it fit. So I put it in a pending tray and got on with the bits of my life that made more sense. It didn't require any effort for me to do this. It just happened. In some ways, it was denial. But denial of what? Of my gut instinct that there was something seriously wrong with me? Perhaps. But everything seemed to conspire against that conclusion. I looked the same – you couldn't see the lump – and I wasn't ill. I had no symptoms as such. It was easy for me to carry on thinking of myself as a healthy person, a robust person as I had always been and as everyone in my family, at that point, had been. Whenever I had to fill in those medical history forms, I never had much to say. And I was, right up until I wasn't, reassured that there was nothing seriously wrong with me.

I can't remember who else I told about the lump and when. All I can remember is the uniform response: don't worry, it won't be anything. Even my GP said so. She told me that whatever the lump was, it wasn't cancer. Cancer didn't feel like this, she said as she examined me. Maybe it was mastitis. I'd had that before, hadn't I, when I was breastfeeding? She gave me a prescription for evening primrose oil and told me to come back the following week if the lump hadn't gone down. *Gone down. How those words echo down the years.* On my way out of the surgery, I found myself making that appointment for the following week. I felt compelled to. It was the same kind of feeling I had had when I discovered the lump. My memory of that feeling is of something muted, but powerful, something intuitive, overriding my natural optimism. I made the appointment for after work, of course.

When I went back to my GP, she suggested I see a specialist, just to be sure. She would write to Charing Cross Hospital where they had a breast unit. I didn't even know where Charing Cross Hospital was. My local hospital, which I can see from my bedroom window, is the Chelsea & Westminster, and the only cancer hospital I'd ever heard of was the Marsden, a ten-minute walk away. Charing Cross Hospital, it seemed, was near Hammersmith, miles away, but she said that it was the right place to go and she knew the consultant, Mr Sinnett. She said they would send me an appointment. I might have to wait a month or so, but no rush. We were just being thorough, after all. There was nothing really to worry about. Then one of those things happened which change everything, but at the time seem insignificant.

'Don't you have health insurance?' she said.

I did, but I'd forgotten. I didn't really approve of it, in the same way that I didn't really approve of private education and in the way that most middle-class liberals don't who have never been seriously tested by the limitations of the NHS and the state school system. My health insurance came with my job. My GP explained that I could see Mr Sinnett privately, that it would make no real difference except that I would probably see him faster and at my own convenience. What persuaded me was the convenience.

I didn't understand the system, so she carefully explained that I would need to ring Mr Sinnett's office and make the appointment myself. She would write a letter of referral. I also needed to check with the insurance company that they were happy with this plan of action. It seemed an awful palaver, but I went along with it. I was offered an appointment for the following week, but I was about to go to Shropshire for half-term and I happily made the appointment for my return: after work, at 7pm, not at Charing Cross after all but at the Cromwell, the private hospital so conveniently halfway between the office and home, where Mr Sinnett held a clinic once a week on a Thursday. I was to have ultrasound a couple of days before – at lunchtime. I was still taking the evening primrose oil. I remember taking it away with me to the cottage. Comical really. And, yes, I did enjoy that holiday. My parents came to visit. The weather was lovely. I slept well.

The Cromwell is a curious place. From the outside it looks like a modern block of flats, all tinted glass and concrete. Inside, it's more like a hotel. The enormous lobby with its opulent beigeness and plants bustles with women in burkas, men in headdresses, and more designer shoes per square foot than Harvey Nicks. The system is simple. If you are having tests, you pay first and claim back later on your insurance. If you are seeing a doctor, you get billed, fast. Either way, you don't get past reception without declaring your financial status and it's hard not to stare at the large bundles of notes carefully counted out by some of the clientele; loadsamonies from another world. I gawped. I, of course, didn't know the system when I went along for my ultrasound, hadn't allowed enough time for the form-filling and bill-paying, and had about £8 in my purse. Luckily I had a credit card, otherwise I'm sure I would have been told to come again another day.

The doctor who carried out the ultrasound said she could see something, wasn't sure what it was, but that Mr Sinnett would look at the scan and see what he thought. I took what she said at face value. I knew there was something there, after all, but I didn't read anything sinister into her vagueness. Now, I'd be vomiting in the corridor. *I know what these bland, evasive comments can mean.*

When I returned to the Cromwell a couple of days later to see Mr Sinnett, I felt jumpy but not half as jumpy as I was for later appointments. Back then, I hadn't got with the programme. I had no clear expectations. I still felt part of the world where maybe bad things happen, but not really bad things. I was also alone. It hadn't occurred to me that I shouldn't be. I was 39. I wasn't in the habit of taking someone with me to the doctor. I have, however, rarely been to a hospital appointment alone since.

There was a nurse in the room when I went in. Mr Sinnett examined me and said there was definitely something there but he needed me to have a mammogram before he could make a proper diagnosis. Three things he needed, he said: ultrasound, an examination and a mammogram. I went into the room next door and had the mammogram. I then sat in the waiting room briefly before the nurse called me back into Mr Sinnett's room. I was sitting, as I said, with my back up against the wall. I was facing Mr Sinnett. To his left was my mammogram, pinned up on some sort of clip. I had seen pictures of breast cancer lumps before, bright white spheres like comets. This was a blurry-looking crescent shape around the top half of my breast. Very large. But it wasn't bright or white, more like static on the TV.

I can see the X-ray clearly now as I write, even though I only saw it that once. What's harder for me to remember is what Mr Sinnett said to me, because as he started to speak, I started to float away. His voice became muffled. I seemed to be looking down at him, at myself, from somewhere near the ceiling. The nurse I hardly registered. One look at her face, full of barely concealed pity, and I turned away from her. I met her again much later. She recognised me. I didn't recognise her. What Mr Sinnett seemed to be saying was that the lump might be cancer, that the area was too large for a biopsy, that I needed to have a quadrantectomy – a what? – so that he could look at the tissue, that if the lump was non-invasive, then that was good, but if it was not, then maybe a mastectomy would be a good idea, then maybe some other treatment, hormonal treatment. I kept asking him to repeat himself. *I couldn't take in anything*. I did manage to ask when I needed to have this quadrant thing done. No rush, said Mr Sinnett. We don't have to do it tomorrow. Next week, maybe early next week, would be fine. Today was Thursday so that sounded like a rush to me. He told me to ring his secretary in the morning to sort out times. He also said I should call my GP and let her know.

Ludicrously, my first thought was that I wasn't sure if I could take the time off work for this operation. I was clinging tenaciously to my old life – what I now see as my old life – a life where *I* decided what extra-curricular activities I had time for. I pressed my health insurance forms on Mr Sinnett. He must sign them. I insisted. It was important. I was fiddling while Rome burned and I knew it. But I didn't know what else to do.

I stumbled out of the room. Mr Sinnett had been kind, gentle with me. But I was plunged into self-pity. I could hardly walk. I staggered through the five-star lobby and out into the street. I found the pedestrian crossing on the Cromwell Road. This is a road, I told myself, a dangerous road: concentrate, wait for the green man. I crossed the road. I walked through the little side street which leads to the Earls Court Road. I crashed into a shop window. *Try and stay upright, I told myself.* Then suddenly I was home.

Kerry had gone home. Simon was there with the children: they were sitting on the sofa. I think Simon was reading them a story, but I'm not sure. I can't remember. I can see them but I can't hear what they are saying. I can remember though that Simon asked me why I was late. I mumbled something about having gone to the hospital for my check-up. He started to ask me how it went – and then abruptly he tuned in, asking me what on earth had happened. The rest of the evening is a blur. I have tried to remember it, but I can't. It may be buried somewhere in my subconscious and I am sure that one day I will be walking along the road thinking about something else entirely and it will suddenly come to me, what happened and how I felt. But for now it's still buried. *All I know is that I didn't scream and that I did sleep.*

There is a notion that when crises happen, we break down, we cry, we wail. Sometimes we do, but often we don't. And when we don't, people remark on how well we are coping. It's nothing to do with coping. It's simply what happens. I had just been told that I might have breast cancer. There was a glimmer of hope – in me, possibly not in Mr Sinnett – that it would be otherwise. Something cataclysmic had happened to me. My sense of myself, my irrational sense of invulnerability and my conviction that I was in charge of my own destiny had been shaken. And yet, in every practical way, nothing had changed at all. I looked the same. My life that evening, in all quotidian detail, was the same. This fact about my health, this 'possible fact' perhaps, was still there. It had not taken over or displaced anything. Yet. *I swung, minute by minute, from feeling floored to feeling normal.* It was hard to know how to react to this ambiguity of feeling, to get the tone right, so my normal good manners prevailed. I couldn't flip a switch and let it all hang out. I would have felt silly.

The next day quickly took on the characteristics of a farce. Kerry came in at nine and Simon and I told her what was happening. She reacted as she would throughout my illness, turning her distress into support, helping to keep the children's lives as normal, as secure, as possible, thereby easing a little the feeling that swept over me then and has never gone away, that I had ruined everything for them.

I can see myself that morning in my white towelling dressing gown, pacing the sitting room. I phoned the office and told my boss, Simon, what had happened and that, as soon as I had fixed up the time for my operation, I would be in. Sorry to be late and all that, I said. He said that I didn't have to go in. Really. I insisted, but he said think about it. It was a typical newspaper conversation, to the point, can-do, but I had, of course, in the chirpiest of ways, gone mad.

I rang my GP. She was on holiday. I was outraged. I took out my anger on the receptionist, practically shouting that I had been told that I might have breast cancer. She asked me if I wanted to see someone else. I couldn't see the point. I then went into private medicine mode. I rang Mr Sinnett's office and organised the operation for the following week, then rang the health insurance company for clearance. The process was oddly bland. You get through to what sounds like a call centre.

'Hi. I think I might have breast cancer,' I said. I gave the person my full name and registration number. I waited while he called up my policy on the computer. 'I need to have a quadrantectomy,' I said. I gave him the details. I had to tell him where it was going to be carried out, and not only who the surgeon was, but the anaesthetist, too.

'Is that OK?' I said, a note of panic entering my voice. 'Am I covered?'

'Yes. That's fine. We'll put the forms in the post. Please remember to get back in touch if you need any more treatment.' *In other words, you may not be covered.* It was over in a couple of minutes, like ordering a toaster from a mail order company. Simon was horrified.

'Do you have to do that yourself?' he said.

I did and, although I didn't know it then, this bizarre exchange would go on and on and on, and not always as satisfactorily. It was slowly dawning on me, however, that I was lucky to have seen Mr Sinnett faster than I would have done on the NHS. Cancer referrals are sometimes fast nowadays, but not always, and I hadn't been considered an urgent case. I would not have been fast-tracked and yet, there I was, with what Mr Sinnett obviously thought was something that needed to be explored urgently.

Later, I became aware of many other benefits to being a private patient. I was lucky in that I would be operated on by Mr Sinnett himself. I wouldn't have been able to specify my surgeon on the NHS and I may have been assigned someone less experienced. I wouldn't necessarily even have had the continuity and reassurance of having consultations with my named consultants either. I would probably have been given appointments with someone I didn't know who would say, as he flicked through my three-inch folder of notes, now which breast did you have the problem with? Other benefits were less important, but helped. I got my own room and bathroom at the hospital. I wasn't disturbed by other patients and had private time with visitors who were allowed to come any time and in any number. There also seemed to be no restrictions on children visiting private rooms. I was, I learned, enormously privileged. Seven years on, I know though that the most important privilege was never having to wait long to see anyone or have any procedure or test. I still wake up in the middle of the night sometimes and wonder what would have happened to me if I had waited for that NHS appointment at Charing Cross, then, as is quite likely, I had cancelled it a few times because of work or home commitments and because it didn't seem urgent. *I also, however, wake up in the middle of the night sometimes and wonder why my health insurance general check-up, six months before I discovered the lump, gave me a clean bill of health.*

That morning I was grappling with a different question. After I had finished my calls, I thought about going into the office. It felt like contemplating going to Mars on a bicycle. I had never felt like this about work before. It was frightening to me. I tried to think about not going to work – my boss had said I didn't need to – but I couldn't imagine that either. I was someone who went to work. I didn't hang around the house. At this point, I didn't have any friends who did either. What on earth was I going to do with myself, I wondered.

Our cleaner Siony arrived. She was surprised to see me. She never saw me. I was always at work when she came. Kerry told her I wasn't well, tried to distract her with titbits about the children. But Siony wasn't thrown off so easily. She isn't daft. She could sense something.

'Have you tried paracetamol?' she said. 'It usually works for me.'

Kerry and I looked at each other. We almost laughed, but only almost. I felt a kind of rage come over me. I was so envious of anyone who could take a paracetamol and feel better that I thought I might cry out. But I didn't, of course.

I decided to go to the gym. Mmm. How puritanical. My body was going haywire and I decide to go to the gym. Was that more fiddling? I think it was probably just pragmatic, some-thing to do. I'd been a member of the Phillimore Club, near the office, for a couple of years. It was a women-only gym and upmarket. When you walked in, you were given a large white towel and a large white towelling robe. There was a small gym, a pool, an exercise room, a sauna, steam room, Jacuzzi and lots of beauty rooms. They served snacks and hot drinks. It was quiet.

The membership was very Kensington, rich older women, quite a few well-heeled fatties. And, crucially, there weren't many blonde-haired bimbos with all-over tans and Gucci handbags, those bizarre creatures who get up every morning and think, 'I look like a Swedish au pair. How absolutely perfect.' I'd been driven out of my local gym by these types when, pale, flabby and with hair like a cavewoman, I'd tried to get back into shape after having Lucian. I couldn't take the competitiveness and didn't go near a gym for years afterwards. When Cosima was born I was tempted by a new gym near work, but was so humiliated by nearly falling off the exercise bike halfway through my induction – the instructor sat me down with one of those sports drinks and paced round me nervously while I 'recovered' – that I only went back twice. It was a huge relief when I found the Phillimore. I was still pale, flabby, although marginally less so, but compared to some of the other members I was way off the bottom rung. Even one of the gym instructors was a bit of a podge, so sometimes I felt like Jamie Lee Curtis in *Perfect*.

My usual routine then was 20 minutes in the gym, twice a week. Although it's probably more accurate to say that 20 minutes in the gym was the routine I aimed for. Sometimes I walked in, collected my towel and robe, showered, sat in the steam room for 10 minutes, ordered a hot chocolate and stretched out on one of the padded benches alongside the pool and slept. If I was lucky, I'd just doze off for 10 minutes. Sometimes, though, I'd fall into a deeper sleep and have to run back to the office.

That morning, I went via the Pan bookshop in the Fulham Road and looked through the health section. There was nothing that seemed to tell me what I wanted to know. But then I didn't really know what I wanted to know. I wanted this thing not to be happening to me. I didn't want to be there looking for books about breast cancer. There was some hippy-dippy stuff, books that told me that, don't worry, most lumps are benign, most women who get breast cancer are over 65. There were pictures of women in cardigans talking about prostheses. *No, no, no.*

I plumped for a book by Miriam Stoppard called *The Breast Book*, a kind of picture book for adults. I took a cab to the gym. When I arrived I felt disorientated again. What was I doing there? I put on my robe. As I was heading for the sauna, I bumped into Sarah, an old friend. After the shortest of hellos, I blurted out that I had a lump which looked bad. Not surprisingly, she looked cornered. She asked me in a staccato voice if I had breastfed the children. Yes, I had. She looked puzzled and told me that it was probably nothing then – this despite the fact that her friend Liz had ovarian cancer and was very ill. She, more than most, knew that the worst can happen. She was in a rush, like I was normally in a rush, and she told me to keep in touch. In fact, she valiantly kept in touch with *me* despite a demanding job and three children. At that precise moment, though, I was left standing alone in the changing room, in my fluffy robe, mirrors all around. *Why do I look the same, I wondered?*

I headed off to the sauna, not daring to look at my body. I couldn't touch my breast, my traitorous breast. I didn't stay long in the heat, just enough to stun me, and then I got my hot chocolate and hid myself away on the bench furthest from the pool. I didn't want anyone to see what I was doing. I felt strangely ashamed as I got out my horribly large book and read.

Most of the book was taken up with breastfeeding, and lumps of the benign type. The chapter on breast cancer was short and matter-of-fact, and reassuring in its simplicity. You find a lump, have it taken out, maybe have some radiotherapy, maybe some chemotherapy and, Bob's your uncle, that's that. I felt better for knowing some of this new language, these words – ductal, lobular, in situ, mastectomy, lumpectomy, radical, modified. It gave me a sense of mastery over my situation. False, of course. But what was I supposed to do with the information I'd been given by Mr Sinnett? And, of course, I was still thinking that everything just might turn out okay, that he was wrong, that I had wasted money on this book, wasted time reading it. I was hoping that I'd soon be looking back on this time and laughing about it, turning it into another anecdote. 'Remember that time I thought I had breast cancer? Wasn't it awful? But thank God it was nothing. Makes you think, though, that kind of thing, doesn't it, shakes you up a bit.'

The weekend was, well, I don't know. I can't remember anything about it except that the children had worms because when I arrived at Charing Cross on the Wednesday for my operation, I had to fill in a number of forms about my medical status – suddenly I had more to write on these forms – and I asked the nurse if I should put down that I might have worms. She didn't think so and obviously thought I was barking. I was still fiddling.

Simon was with me and then my parents arrived. We sat there, trying to make conversation. I was in the private wing of the hospital, the 15th floor as it was usually, rather unimaginatively, called, and I had my own room with chairs and a coffee table. We ordered tea and biscuits. Then Mr Sinnett arrived. He quietly and carefully went over what the operation would entail

– taking away a quarter of my breast which would then be examined. I asked him what he thought he would find. He said that he thought it probably was cancer, but that he could never say for sure until he had a lab report. We had moved on. *The news had got worse.* Mr Sinnett was holding my hand and walking me into the cancer world, one step at a time, with careful words. So that's how it's done, I thought. A slight change of emphasis here, a new word there, and there you were, somewhere else. Right then I had suddenly moved from possibly to probably.

Mr Sinnett is apparently Welsh, but I never absorb this kind of information about people. He obviously doesn't go around the place calling people boyo, but there is, I'm told, a slight inflection in his voice. I'm aware of something, but I tend to use a different set of criteria to place people, in the way that all English people like to place others. My method is just as narrow and judgemental, but has nothing to do with accent, looks, success, which school someone went to, who their father is. It's everything to do with intelligence. Not qualifications, but a way of looking at the world. And it's everything to do with humour. Not jokes, but a certain self-deprecation. Mr Sinnett is both clever and self-deprecating, so I felt that despite my predicament I was one lucky bunny. If I'd met Mr Sinnett at a party, I would have been thrilled. Sadly, this was a poor substitute for a party, but I was still pleased to have him there. At some point, my friend Paula did some research on him and pronounced him an excellent surgeon, too, but I never felt I needed any confirmation of his talents, a second opinion. I instinctively felt safe with him.

I asked for a pre-med. There had to be some perks. But they didn't seem to do pre-meds. Simon walked down to theatre with me. As I went through the swinging double doors into . . . into knowledge, I suppose, Mr Sinnett took my hand and said everything would be fine; then the anaesthetic rushed through my body, one of the most wonderful sensations in the world.

I don't have much to say about surgery. They knock you out, they chop you up, they sew you up and then you wake up. In pain. Perhaps feeling sick. It's always the same. The only thing that matters is that the surgeon knows what they are doing. I stayed in hospital for two nights and then went home wearing a plaster and feeling sore. I made an appointment to see Mr Sinnett the following Monday when the results on the lab tests would be ready. This time, I was to go to Parkside hospital in Wimbledon, in the early evening. You get around when you go private.

So I waited. The most vivid memory of that wait is the hours leading up to the appointment. I went to Pizza Express in the Fulham Road, the one with the Sixties psychedelic decor. Kerry was taking the children for a treat and I tagged along. I found I had to concentrate to do the simplest of tasks, to listen to what people were saying. My mind wasn't elsewhere, it was nowhere. I also felt sick. When Simon got back from work, we drove to the hospital. We had to wait a while. This isn't supposed to happen when you go private, I thought. Mr Sinnett apologised for the wait and said that he had only just got the results from the lab. *And then he told me that I had cancer.*

What did I say? Something along the lines of you've got to help me, I can't die, I've got two young children. Please. Please. I was back up on the ceiling and when I try to envisage this meeting, it sounds as muffled as the first, heavy. But I didn't cry, I didn't collapse or faint.

I had an unusual type of breast cancer apparently – lobular. Ductal is more common. There wasn't as much information about lobular, they didn't see it often. The only relevant fact seemed to be that it didn't appear to affect the other breast which I didn't even know was a consideration. The tumour was large though and the edges ill-defined, so it was probably on the move, spreading. My best bet was to have a mastectomy. Somehow I managed to discuss this. Why could I not have a lumpectomy? Everything I'd ever heard about breast cancer seemed to suggest that mastectomies were a thing of the past, old school, unnecessarily radical, possibly even sexist. There was talk about achieving a safe margin round the tumour, how much of my breast would be destroyed anyway. All things considered, Mr Sinnett thought a mastectomy would be safer. Simon asked him what he would recommend for his own wife. Mastectomy, he said.

The best – yes, in the world of cancer, there are such things, there is a hierarchy of awfulness, bad luck – type of breast cancer to have is, apparently, ductal carcinoma in situ. It's not on the move, so you can whip it out, have some radiotherapy and are quite possibly cured. I was already in a different category, but it wasn't yet clear which of the bad categories I would end up in.

Mr Sinnett explained that, at the same time as the mastectomy, he would remove the lymph nodes in my right armpit to ascertain whether the cancer was spreading, as seemed likely given the ill-defined edges. When breast cancer spreads, he explained, it hits the lymph nodes first and the extent to which they are affected, if they are, determines the next line of treatment, perhaps chemotherapy, perhaps hormone treatment.

Some surgeons, he said, sampled lymph nodes – took out a few and extrapolated from what they found. He preferred to look at them all. I may have looked as if I was listening, but I was only half-listening. I understood in a technical sense the lymph-node issue, but, quite wrongly, I thought it was a side-issue, relevant to some cases, but not mine. Hormone therapy went over my head as I didn't know what it was. In my shock and ignorance, I stuck on the two words I could just about understand: mastectomy and chemotherapy. I felt like I was at the entrance to a long, dark tunnel. Mr Sinnett was trying to persuade me to go in, perhaps to the light at the other end. But I didn't want to go in, my mind wouldn't let me and there seemed little evidence that there was any light at the other end. When I asked if I would be okay if I had all this treatment, Mr Sinnett told me, quite truthfully, that he didn't know. Nobody knew what would happen to me, he said. I couldn't respond. I was shocked all over again. *Why the hell couldn't he give me some reassurance, I thought. This is 1997, not 1907.* I must have asked him what hormone therapy meant though because he started to tell me that it was a way of switching off my ovaries. *What?*

An image then came unbidden into my head, a Hollywood image, of the Alien bursting out of John Hurt's chest. It was accompanied by the loud ticking of a clock. And suddenly I wanted my cancer out. Now. I couldn't see the tunnel any more. The word mastectomy became as nothing. I was leapfrogging over it to another place, another time, when I would not be contaminated. Chemotherapy and hormone therapy? I didn't give them another thought. *Bring on the knives, I silently screamed.*

But if that makes it sound as though I were spoiling for a fight, ready for action, it is only half the story. I found it difficult to walk back to the car. I found it hard to speak. A part of me was dead and buried already, my children orphans. I was crushed by the weight of the idea that cancer equals death.

It's hard now to appreciate how little I knew about cancer back then. Simon knew more. His father had died of lung cancer when he was 12. His mother had also had breast cancer. He has vivid memories of his father's illness, wheeling home the cylinders of oxygen for him to use at home. The clearest memory he has of his mother's illness is of standing in the hospital car park and waving to her as she waved at him through a window. Children were not allowed on the wards in those days. His mother did not die of her breast cancer. She survived, but she never spoke of it, not to her children, or me. The mastectomies in those days were radical, the radiotherapy vicious, but she never said anything. Cancer was part of Simon's childhood and he was tired of its sadness and had, he thought, escaped from it with me and my family, so healthy and robust, as yet untouched.

My own experience of cancer was minimal. My uncle had died of asbestosis when I was a teenager and my paternal grandmother had died of stomach cancer when I was in my early thirties. But other family deaths were of the ripe-old-age variety and relatively peaceful. I was a beginner when it came to cancer and death, perhaps more than most. When I became a mother, I worried more about death, about how I could be mown down by a car. I felt more vulnerable, but I wasn't preoccupied with it. I never made a will.

The only event which had shaken me out of this slumber, albeit momentarily, was the death from leukaemia of my friend

Lindsay's husband when I was in my thirties. They had a daughter, Ellie, and Lindsay was pregnant with their second child, Hope, when he died. I heard the news from a colleague when I was walking into work at the *Sunday Times* one morning. He ambled up to me and said, '*You* know Lindsay, John's wife, don't you?' I said I did and then he told me. I went into my office, shut the door, cried, rang Lindsay, said a few hopeless things, got on with my work and decided that I should have another baby. Lucian was, at this point, a toddler and Simon and I had always planned to have another child, but had been havering, waiting for some mythical perfect time to get pregnant. Now there seemed no point in waiting. You never knew what was round the corner, I thought, so *carpe diem*.

But I never seriously thought anything *was* waiting round any corner for me, so now I felt nothing but utter disbelief mixed with a terrible, debilitating fatalism. When we arrived back home that evening, the children were asleep and Kerry was waiting for us. Simon told her what had happened and she was distraught and kind, proclaiming that these things always happened to good people. She said she would do everything she could to help. I didn't know then but I was to hear these words from many other people over the coming months, but they rarely translated into action. Kerry kept her word and more.

Simon rang my parents, but I could not speak and when they rang back later, they were rendered inarticulate, too. I sat on the edge of the sofa, repeating *ad nauseam* how I couldn't believe what was happening to me. Then Simon changed the record for me.

'You can't turn the clock back,' he said. 'This has happened and we now have to deal with it. And we will.'

It was a verbal slap in the face, but rallied me. Doors had been slamming noisily around me, the doors which led to my future, but Simon was opening one. The outlook was bleak, but this is what we could do, we could face it, head on. The shock of my diagnosis had catapulted him back into his childhood world of cancer, that world with no guarantees and, this time, with the possibility of not only being left again, but being left with two children to bring up. Yet somehow a certain fearlessness had kicked in, too, overriding his dismay, which enabled him to help me in a way which no one else has ever been able to. I don't know where he found the strength for what he did that evening or the months and years ahead. It was and is, to me, a miracle. I am a whining, self-pitying child on a long and difficult walk and he has held my hand tight, dragging me through the undergrowth, untangling me from the briars, insisting that, no, these thistles are not impassable, this ditch is not too wide to jump, and, yes, we are nearly there.

I'm still not sure exactly where it is we are going and, on that terrible evening, I had no thoughts of the journey ahead. I was simply grateful to Simon. I have no idea what we talked about, but I do know that there was no need to talk about the treatment. Simon was as sure as I was that I should have the mastectomy, however grotesque and imperfect an option it seemed. We could not reject it. I know of people who resist and struggle and fight against conventional medicine. They talk about ancient systems of healing, harnessing the body's natural powers. It's romantic, soft-focus stuff. For me, it has always seemed, at best, harmless, a pleasant complement to conventional treatment which makes people feel they are doing something for themselves, but it's no substitute and it seems

31

peevish to reject all modern medicine. It's like refusing to grow up and I've never seen any good come of it.

It's hard being sensible and grown-up when all you want to do is hide under the bedclothes and have someone bring you a hot water bottle, some tea and toast, a couple of paracetamol and perhaps some echinacea which will sort everything out while you rest up listening to *Desert Island Discs*. It's not that hard, though. When, that evening, I faced up to what I needed to do to save my life, I shut down, shut down my emotions. I couldn't make sense of them, they seemed too huge, incontinent. They felt like vampires, sucking out my life blood, so I blocked them, repressed them, in order to get on with the business in hand. It was a version of what had happened to me when I first found the lump in my breast, but this time it truly was denial as I now had some facts to deny. As one of my doctors said later though, 'Don't knock denial. It can be very useful.'

It is, but it is much misunderstood. It's often talked about as though it is a form of psychological death that we indulge in at our peril. But it is in fact an involuntary response. I didn't decide to go into denial. It pretty much just happened as I became overwhelmed – and it got me through, sort of. I suddenly couldn't have cared less about the meaning of cancer, the meaning of life, the bigger picture. All I wanted to do was concentrate on making myself safe. The angst, the navel-gazing would come later. In spades. As it does for many and, I think, should. For although denial works wonders in the short-term, it's dangerous when it goes on and on. When the crisis is past, it seems to have diminishing returns as a strategy and, rather than being involuntary, requires ever greater resources of energy to maintain. Emotionally, you go into the red. But I didn't know any of this back then. I simply found myself putting away thoughts of life and death and the future, and concentrated on the detail, looking for God, I suppose.

In this foggy, muted state, I bumbled along organising my operation. There was no immediate rush, said Mr Sinnett, and there was a slot two weeks hence. I became obsessed with the idea that the cancer had not yet spread to my lymph nodes but would do so during this period. I could almost feel it spreading, a fantastical idea, but exactly what I felt.

I had decided to have a reconstruction at the same time as my mastectomy and lymph node clearance – I thought it would make me feel better and I also wanted to avoid a third round of surgery – so Mr Sinnett recommended that I go and see Mr Searle, a reconstructive surgeon. I saw him at the Lister Hospital near Chelsea Bridge. As with Mr Sinnett, I struck lucky. I liked him enormously. He was informal, relaxed and greeted me by kissing me on both cheeks. Later, I discovered that most of the nurses adored him. He told me what to expect – you can't recreate a natural breast exactly, especially if that breast belongs to a 39-year-old woman who has had two children – but he would do his best. I would probably have to have surgery on the other breast to make them match, but that could wait. He also told me that although I now felt self-conscious about taking off my top and letting strangers stare at my breasts, after a while I wouldn't give a damn.

Then, much to my surprise, he talked to me about the emotional upheaval of having cancer. He scribbled a diagram on the corner of a piece of paper which I still have. I didn't fully understand its significance at the time, but it has turned out to be entirely accurate. The diagram looked like what you see on those heart monitors on *ER*. There was a straight line with a second line running through it, depicting a range of mountains above the line, chasms below. At the beginning of the line, the peaks and troughs were dramatic and close together. Further along, they became shallower and gentler. Mr Searle said that being diagnosed with cancer was like being hit by a truck. You were stunned. Then your emotions went haywire, way up and way down. Gradually, over time, the highs and lows would become more manageable. He never said they would peter out.

A month earlier, I had never met a surgeon, and now I had met two. They seemed to me extraordinary. I once asked Mr Sinnett if he worked long hours. He said no, he had an easy time of it. He said he worked regular hours. (This was at around 7.30 in the morning as I was waking up in my hospital bed.) He liked to do his rounds early in the morning, he said. When I had seen him at Parkside Hospital, he would have finished up at around 9pm. Office hours were taken up by clinics and operations. Saturdays, he said, he only did rounds and was usually home for lunch. His answer made me feel small, petty.

I was also fascinated by Mr Sinnett's and Mr Searle's ability to go, more often than not, where no one had gone before. I have tried to imagine what it feels like to stand over someone and cut into their flesh and rummage around, what it feels like to have the power to destroy or heal, sometimes the latter being a result of the former. Did they have off days? Did they have days when they were coasting, when they'd had a late night or broken sleep with a new baby? It didn't seem possible or acceptable. I have also tried to imagine what it feels like to have someone like me stare into your eyes and beg for help. How do you get up every morning and face that responsibility? How do you protect yourself? How do you stop yourself thinking that maybe, just maybe, you are God? No wonder some surgeons are weird, arrogant, off-hand, revel in the language of the battlefield. A friend who has written a lot about the health service sums up some of the doctors he has met as brutish rugger-buggers who like shagging nurses. I felt lucky. Mr Sinnett and Mr Searle were unfailingly civilised.

While I was waiting for my mastectomy, I had another stroke of luck, the significance of which I only understood later. Mr Sinnett sent me for bone and liver scans, and a chest X-ray. I trotted off to the Cromwell again. The chest X-ray was straightforward, the liver scan a quick whoosh of ultrasound. The bone scan was scarier. I was taken into a room with the equivalent of a skull and crossbones on the door, and injected with something to light up my bones. I was then told to go away for a couple of hours to let it work its Ready-Brek magic – and, by the way, the nurse said, don't go cuddling your children tonight. The scan itself was slow but painless and I went home, trying to oh-so-casually not cuddle and kiss my little children to protect them from my toxic rays. But this, in my ignorance, was the sum total of my distress.

When I got the results, the scans were clear. I was pleased but not nearly as pleased as I should have been. I didn't expect them to show anything. I was persisting in thinking that breast cancer appeared, well, in the breast. I had neither fully addressed the lymph node issue nor taken in – or perhaps had chosen not to take in – that the bones, liver and lungs are where breast cancer is most likely to spread, metastasise, and that these scans would tell Mr Sinnett if that had already happened. If it had, then my prognosis would have been even grimmer.

My reaction when I went back to Charing Cross to have the stitches from my quadrantectomy taken out was off the mark, too. As he examined me, Mr Sinnett said he could feel the lymph nodes in my armpit. He said it might be a reaction to the operation – or not. I didn't question this observation. It had too much of that tunnel about it. *Now I'd be interrogating him, mentally fast-forwarding to my funeral.*

Or perhaps not. I am an asker, a seeker of information. I always want to know exactly what is going on and the best way to deal with problems. Or I did. When it came to my cancer, the asking came and went, and still does. The dance, the dance in which everyone knows that there's only one real question – am I going to die? – is hard to bear. So sometimes I asked many questions. My mother rather optimistically once suggested that soon I'd know more than the doctors. Other times, I said nothing. I don't remember saying much to other people either. How do you ring up someone and say, Hi, I've got cancer. Calls from other people were difficult, too, having to answer a casual how-are-you with a casual well-I've-got-cancer. But soon the bad news got out and the phone started ringing with callers who knew what was up, and the cards and flowers started arriving, every day. It was wonderful. I never realised I had so many friends. As my friend Paula said, the tom-toms had sounded.

During this period, I went back to work. I was embarrassed by the time I had already taken off – two weeks. But just as I felt I was getting on top of things, I got a call telling me that due to coordination problems between the schedules of Mr Sinnett and Mr Searle, my operation had been brought forward, to the next day. I was to be the first operation, so I should report to Charing Cross that evening. I had to rush home and pack. I was angry. *My life, my old orderly life, was spiralling further and further out of control.*

I duly reported to Charing Cross with Simon. I was back on the 15th floor. The room had a view, of the river and the Harrods storerooms. I could almost see the River Café, a tantalising glimpse of another kind of world, of glamorous birthday treats, so near yet so far. The room stank and was hot. Something was waiting to be fixed. It made me unbearably cross. I wanted it fixed, now, immediately. I became a hoity-toity harridan. It was fixed. My mother suddenly appeared. She had travelled all the way from Essex, a three-hour round trip.

Mr Sinnett swung by to draw on my chest. I felt like one of those cut-out paper dollies. Cut here, here and here. We discussed lopping off a mole while he was at it. He said I shouldn't wash the area. This irritated me, too. It was a pattern that was to repeat itself over the coming months. Not being able to make sense of the bigger picture and concentrating on the detail, the here and now, made me disproportionately angry about the detail – I suppose it was just the bigger, more terrifying, picture breaking through briefly before melting away again. I've seen this reaction in other people, too, people *in extremis*. They react strongly to some seemingly minor discomfort, something which in the grand scheme of things is nothing. The detail in this case was that I couldn't have a normal bath, which felt undignified. I had a careful shower, a small gesture of defiance, a desperate gesture of normality. The anaesthetist came to see me and I banged on and on about how he had, absolutely had, to make sure that I was asleep. I was obsessed with the stories floating around at the time of people who had been awake during operations, feeling the knives cutting into them, unable to signal for help. I demanded a sleeping tablet and slept.

In fact, I slept fairly well throughout my illness. I slept heavily at times, my body and mind gleefully escaping from the terror of my daily life. Sometimes I would wake in the night with tears on my face, but I always went back to sleep again, and I have no memories of any dreams during this period, apart from one, the most terrifying dream I have ever had, much later on. I found this odd as I had always dreamed vividly. As a child, I had nightmares, I was a sleepwalker and, although the nightmares diminished when I started living with Simon, they were a normal part of my life. Now I think that I probably was dreaming – it seems, according to the people I have asked, to be impossible to sleep dreamlessly, to close the Freudian royal road – so I probably blanked out these dreams. *I had enough nightmares to face in my waking hours.*

The nurses woke me early the next morning, earlier than I'd been told. I was given a gown and elasticated stockings to put on. Mr Sinnett popped his head round the door and told me he would see me in the operating theatre. Then, briefly, I was on my own. I started to panic that I would be taken down to theatre before Simon arrived. I tried to think of something to do to distract myself, prepare myself, but there was nothing to do. I brushed my teeth and sat, expectant and miserable, on the bed.

I felt overwhelmed by loneliness. Then, suddenly, a porter appeared and just as I was about to be wheeled out, Simon rushed in and he came down to theatre with me. He held my hand and I started crying, very quietly. He kissed me as we reached the swinging doors and then I could see Mr Sinnett and, beyond him, some other people in their scrubs, waiting. Mr Sinnett held my hand and told me he liked to listen to Classic FM while he worked. He smiled at me and then the anaesthetic kicked in. Bliss.

My memories of the following days are vague, but unpleasant. I awoke from the five-hour operation to a feeling of enormous pressure. It felt as though there was a heavy weight on my chest. I tried to move, perhaps to sit up, I'm not entirely sure what I was trying to do, but I couldn't do anything, I couldn't move. I was terrified. Then I became aware of someone next to me, a nurse. She was telling me that she had had breast cancer and that since her treatment she had had a child and was fine. I have no idea who she was, but she was kind and gentle with me. She also spoke to me in a way that I have come to recognise over the years as the voice of experience, the voice of someone who has been there. It's almost impossible to describe how that voice differs from the voice of ordinary empathy, but it does. There is a cutting to the chase, a clarity. The voice says, let's not fuck around here, let's talk about what matters. It's the embrace that a mother gives a small child who has woken in the night after a bad dream.

When I was wheeled back into my room, Simon was there with my parents. I had one of those clicker things to administer morphine as and when I needed it. I drifted in and out of sleep, clicking and clicking and clicking. My right arm seemed to be strapped to my chest. There were three drains coming out of my chest and back, tubes emptying gruesome-looking gunk into plastic bottles. I still couldn't move. I had to pee lying down, the weirdest of sensations. I felt sick and had something injected into my bottom. Sometimes I thought I was hallucinating.

A couple of days later a nurse insisted that I get up and wash myself in the bathroom. Up until then I had been bed-bathed. I hated her, but found I could do it. I looked in the bathroom mirror. I looked the same. Except for my eyes that is. They belonged to someone else, someone in a horror movie who has just heard the madman coming up the stairs.

After another couple of days I was feeling much better, sitting in a chair, eating, reading, receiving visitors. Simon was there all the time as far as I can remember. The children came with Kerry who must have been working round the clock to free up Simon. My family came. My friend Anita came, slogging across London heavily pregnant in the oppressive summer heatwave. My friend Paula came, unannounced, rushing in on Saturday morning with a copy of *Martha Stewart Living* magazine and making me laugh. My oldest friend Anna, the best dancing partner I ever had, who was living in Paris, rang every day. It helped. Mr Sinnett and Mr Searle monitored my progress.

Every now and then I'd walk round the 15th floor in a feeble attempt to get moving. I hauled round the drains in a sturdy, brightly coloured carrier bag from the clothes shop Voyage. One by one they were removed and then Mr Searle appeared, to take off my dressings. He asked me to look at myself, to touch my reconstructed breast. I was nervous, but not overly. I had, I felt, simply done what had to be done. But it looked much better than I had imagined, which I suppose had been a half-grapefruit stuck on to an ironing board, some kind of Sarah Lucas-style installation. I was pleased. Then he explained that what I was feeling, I was feeling in my fingertips. There was no feeling in the breast. It was disconcerting. He also told me that I needed to start moving my arm more, that whenever he saw me I had it clutched to my chest like a bird with a broken wing. I was completely unaware that I had been doing this.

I asked to see a physio, but she wasn't much help. When I showed her a leaflet of post-operative exercises published by Breast Cancer Care that I'd got from the gym, she asked me how she could get hold of it. Then, all at once, I was ready to go home, much earlier than the 10 days I had been told to expect. How strong I was, how amazing was my recovery.

Something else had happened during my stay though. About halfway through, the lab results came through on my lymph nodes. Mr Sinnett gave them to me on one of his early morning rounds. I awoke to see him standing there and, with his hand gently touching my arm, he told me that a high number were affected and therefore I should have chemotherapy because, although the scans had shown nothing, there were probably cancer cells circulating in my body. The chemo would blast them. A colleague, he said, Professor Coombes, would stop by and talk me through the treatment. It was more bad news, but I found it hard to react. Each step of the way through my diagnosis when there had been two possible outcomes, I had been dealt the worst outcome. My lump was not benign. It was not in situ. It was not possible for me to have a lumpectomy. My lymph nodes were affected. I went back to sleep.

Professor Coombes came to see me later that day, rushing in wearing a white coat and a stethoscope. Mr Sinnett and Mr Searle had always been dressed in civvies when they weren't in scrubs. I had been told that his bedside manner was quite different from theirs as well, so had been expecting the worst kind of brute. But although he was matter-of-fact, not a hand-holder or a kisser, he was charming and I was entranced. He was like no one I had ever met before, a scientist, a dealer in facts and formulas. In journalism, slivers of information are turned into 800-word features and published in newspapers and magazines. Someone somebody in the office knows is selling their second home. Hey presto. It's a trend. Second homes are so over. Professor Coombes, I quickly learned, would have to be practically buried in statistics and facts before he would come to even the most tentative of conclusions. It made for some amusing misunderstandings.

This meeting was not funny though. I knew nothing about chemotherapy, what it was or how it was administered. I just had the idea that it was the worst the medical profession could throw at you. What I quickly discovered was that it was the best the medical profession can throw at you despite the fact that, as I was to discover, it is imprecise. Yet again, there were no guarantees that it would destroy all the possible cancer cells in my body. That was the aim, but not the promise.

Professor Coombes was obviously used to people like me, clueless. He explained, clearly and carefully, that he was running a trial for a treatment called a peripheral stem cell transplant which might – he took great pains to emphasise the might – be more effective than the current standard treatment. It was, as I understood it, a way of giving patients a higher dose of chemotherapy from which they would normally find it hard, perhaps impossible, to recover, the point being that more chemotherapy might – might, might, might – equal more life. Baldly speaking, the treatment would involve a short course of standard chemotherapy in outpatients, then the high-dose chemotherapy in hospital. In between, some of my stem cells – mother cells – would be collected and frozen. Then, after the high-dose chemotherapy, I would be given back these stem cells to help me recover from its effects – baldly speaking, the destruction of my immune system. This hospital bit would take about a month. Baldly speaking, it wasn't very nice. The alternative was standard chemotherapy, seven months in outpatients. Not nice either, but not so not very nice as the stem cell transplant. I had to choose.

I tried a different tack. 'Do I really have to have chemotherapy?'

'No, it's up to you. You can go home now if you want.'

This took me by surprise. 'But what do you think?'

'I think,' Professor Coombes said, looking me straight in the eye, 'that there are three stages of cancer. In the first, we can probably cure you. In the second, we hope we can help you. In the third, we try to keep you comfortable. At the moment, you are in the second category.'

At the moment? What would you choose? 'I'll have the chemotherapy,' I said. 'And the high-dose.'

'I'll send up a nurse to explain it all to you.'

And off he went. I never gave my decision another thought. Even when, years later, the results from the trial seemed to suggest that high-dose chemotherapy was no better than standard – they are still being studied – I never for a moment regretted what I agreed to. I trusted Professor Coombes and I wanted a crack at the best chance of survival, however tentative it seemed. I would also do it again, if that was what was on offer, even though it was the most harrowing experience of my life and I hated every single second of it. Later, much later, I read an article in *The New Yorker* describing the treatment as the killing cure, which seemed about right, apart from the cure bit.

3

May You Never

Chemotherapy. Chemo. The poison bit of slash, poison and burn, those unlovely treatment options for cancer. This is how they do it. You sit in a chair and you proffer your arm, the inside of your arm. They – this nurse, that nurse – look at your arm carefully, for a good vein. (This, at first, is the easy part. Later it gets to be the worst part or perhaps one of the worst parts.) They then insert a cannula, a little tube, into the vein, which is then attached to whatever is hanging on the drip stand next to you and they start pumping highly toxic chemicals into your body. Sometimes, they do it by hand, too, with one of those syringes they give you with children's medicines. The chemicals are injected in a specific, almost sacred, order and at different speeds. It doesn't hurt, but it is boring. My cocktail was called FEC and took, on average, three hours to administer. Other drugs were pumped into me, too – anti-emetics and steroids. It's a surprisingly simple procedure, chemotherapy, and this simplicity threw me off my guard briefly. *How can something so simple be so bad?*

I was scheduled to have five sessions in outpatients at Charing Cross, spread over three months. Then, after a short break, I would go into the Hammersmith Hospital for the peripheral stem cell transplant. The five sessions of standard chemo were, I knew, considered to be the easy part of the protocol, a mere warm-up, adding to my confusion about just how bad this experience was going to be.

Other people had no doubts about what chemo was going to be like – the pits – but they seemed to find it hard to get a handle on it, too. Some asked if I felt sick, which I expected and could answer easily. But the question I was most often asked was what the initials FEC stood for, usually by people who had no real need for the information, but somehow felt that having it, maybe even just asking for it, signalled engagement with my treatment, empathy. The trouble was I couldn't tell them what they wanted to know. I knew what the initials stood for, I'd been given this information, but I was never able to remember it. Most of the time, FEC simply reminded me of *Father Ted*. The serious information slithered around in my brain like mercury, ungraspable. It seemed, I suppose, to be beside the point. What I could remember about the chemicals was that the E one was the worst, the most poisonous, and was red. Also that one of the other drugs made my bottom feel prickly, which was possibly too much information for most people.

The point about the chemo for me was that I was required to be awake and therefore participate in the ritual, chat to the nurse as she sat with me on and off through those hours, as she pumped the poison into my body. This participation had been a notional idea during the first part of my treatment. The tests had not been that unpleasant and relatively quick, and I'd been asleep during the surgery, the bits that seemed against nature and almost, but unfortunately not quite, unimaginable. *I never actually saw the knives.* With the chemotherapy, however, a different attitude prevailed. 'You're in John Wayne country now' seemed to be about the measure of it. The most unhinging aspect was that proffering of my arm, not once, but repeatedly. It conjured up images of concentration camps, of doors closing, of unspeakable choices to be made, and made, however perversely, willingly.

I wasn't so mired in self-pity that I couldn't see the melodrama in this image, that I was not fully aware of the fact that I was not actually a victim of genocide, merely a victim of an imperfect science. But there was something about the beseeching eyes of those inhabitants of concentration camps that I had seen on newsreels that floated into my mind every time I proffered my arm, willingly. I'm not sure that anyone noticed though. Most of the time, I chatted away quite normally. It wasn't that I was pretending to feel fine when I wasn't. It was just that these feelings appeared like flashes of lightning, disappearing as fast as they appeared out of the numbness. I couldn't get hold of them and I certainly didn't know how to express them at the time. It seemed irrelevant, ungrateful even, to complain. I was silenced by my new place in the world. The priority was saving my body. My soul would have to wait. So I kept quiet, kept my disturbed mind to myself.

The routine of my chemo never varied. My appointments were on Mondays. I would arrive around 9am, have a blood test – go to bloods as they say – then see Professor Coombes, who would decide by looking at my blood count if I was up to having the chemo, an integral part of chemo's machismo. You may have to be dying to be offered it, but you can't get it if you are too weak. He would then write a prescription for the chemo which would vary slightly according to the blood count, sometimes full strength, sometimes not. I was never, thankfully, told that I couldn't have it at all, but I was told that this tended to happen to younger patients more. I would then go up to the 15th floor, the private wing, and sit in one of the rooms. I usually sat on the bed – very much the professional patient – and Simon sat on the chair. We would watch TV, read, or pretend to. Then, when the drugs arrived, which could sometimes take hours, I would be cannulated and I would have the chemo. I would go home late afternoon, if I was lucky.

After the first session, I stayed in hospital overnight to be monitored in case I had a severe reaction. I didn't in the sense that I didn't instantly go into a coma, throw up or whatever unspecified horror could be termed a severe reaction, but I did experience what I wrongly thought was a delayed reaction to the chemo and the meal I ate that evening.

The chemo took about four hours to go through that first time because my veins recoiled from the E drug, which slowed down the process. Who could blame them? Afterwards, I waited to start vomiting, but I felt good, not ill. I was naïvely triumphant. I had done it. And I was hungry. The nurse had said that the sickness often kicked in later, but I wasn't really listening. It didn't make any kind of sense and I tucked into an Indian vegetarian rice dish which I enjoyed. It was light and fragrant, perfect for a warm evening. I then read my book and slept, well. I went home the next morning feeling smug. I started feeling sick on the Wednesday. It was, in hindsight, not so bad really, but I couldn't do anything except lie still. The thought of food was repellent, specifically anything resembling the food I had eaten that night. Indeed, for about four years, I couldn't eat Indian food at all. The mere smell of it was enough to make me feel queasy. The one time I did eat it, at my friend Jane's party, I threw up all night. I can eat it now, but I wouldn't choose to. I also cannot bear the smell of the perfume I wore at this time. Smells seem to take a shortcut through my brain, providing me with instant and total recall of those chemotherapy sessions. There are other triggers, madeleines, but all the memories are unpleasant. For years, I would feel nauseous just walking through the doors of the hospital.

After that first chemo session, my reaction followed the same pattern. For the first 24 hours after the treatment, I'd think I'd got away with it, thought I was special. Then a day later I'd start feeling nauseous, so much so that I often went to bed. I was never actually sick – that would have been a relief – but I couldn't eat and wallowed in self-pity. It was like morning sickness in pregnancy in that it had nothing to do with mornings and everything to do with dragging myself round feeling bad, really bad. And, as when I was pregnant, I sipped Coke and nibbled on digestive biscuits. I also, though, took powerful drugs for the nausea so I presume I would have felt much worse without them, but the words 'sail through' never became part of my chemo vocabulary. The nausea would last a couple of days and then I would feel fine. Fine as in the kind of fine you feel after a terrible hangover, battered but optimistic, weak but triumphal. Briefly though.

The process wore me down. Familiarity did not breed contempt and ignorance did turn out to have been a kind of bliss. The more I knew about chemotherapy, the more sessions

I had, the weedier I became. There were problems. After a while, it was hard to find a good vein and my veins became intelligent, jumped out of the way as the cannula came for them, so getting cannulated became difficult. Once it took three hours. Every now and then, a different nurse would arrive to 'have a go'. It made me cry in the end. Not the pain: that was bearable. But the hopelessness of the situation. Eventually I was sent down to the NHS chemo suite. Suite? Whoever came up with that? One of the old hands, as she was referred to, cannulated me in seconds, painlessly. I hadn't realised that there was a hierarchy in the world of cannulation and that the nurses on the 15th floor weren't necessarily old hands, so I demanded that, in future, I be cannulated in the chemo suite before retiring up to the 15th floor to have my chemo. It was another Violet Elizabeth Bott moment, which still makes me cringe.

I was also unnerved by what was described as the harvesting – such a sweet, pastoral description – of my white blood cells which would be frozen in preparation for the transplant. After my first chemo session, I had to arrange for a nurse to visit me every morning for a week to inject me with GCSF, a drug which would make these cells proliferate. The hospital wanted lots. The injection was fine, the effects were not. I experienced what is called bone pain. It was a pain which seemed to be deep inside me and ran down my leg from my hip. My automatic response was to pull my knees into my chest. It made no difference and it felt like a pain that no drug could reach. I found it hard to stand up. Then when I went into the hospital for the actual harvest, I had a central line put in. This is a long tube which is poked through your neck and re-emerges in your chest. Attached to it are various ports through which you can be injected without being cannulated – useful for long-term chemo – or, in my case, through which your white blood cells can be siphoned off.

I reported to the hospital in the morning, desperate for pain relief for the bone pain. It seemed to take ages to organise. I walked around the room, goose-stepping in an ineffectual attempt to relieve the pain. Then I was given a broad spectrum antibiotic to prepare me for the line. I felt hot and when I told Simon, he looked up from his newspaper and was horrified. I looked like I was burning up. My reaction to the antibiotic was called – very technical this – red man syndrome. Then I had the line put in. It was horrible. They give you a local anaesthetic and guide in the tube by looking at a screen. You can look, too, if you want. I didn't. The people who do it may be technical wizards but they have the bedside manner you imagine Margaret Thatcher might have had. They talk among themselves, about what they are looking at on the screen and what they are doing that evening. You are of interest purely as a technical problem. So you lie there like a lump of meat – you mustn't move – and you feel so lonely that you want to cry. And what makes it worse is that, just like with the chemo, you know you have agreed to this repellent procedure. It feels, I suppose, humiliating.

I stayed in hospital overnight and the next day I had my cells harvested, a completely painless procedure overseen by the nurse who Professor Coombes had sent up to explain my treatment to me. She was quietly efficient and had generously dealt with the health insurance company when they balked at paying for the stem cell treatment – later, I saw why. The bills for my treatment came to around £70,000. She hooked me up to a machine and the cells were, well, harvested. Then when she had checked that she had enough, the line was taken out. She asked me to look away and then cough. As I coughed, she pulled it out, covered in gunk. Grotesque, but painless. She was a pro and I felt bereft when she left later that summer.

I often felt during this period – quite wrongly as it turned out – that I had reached rock bottom, that I was living in a parallel universe which was a negative of what I thought of as the normal world. I tried, I really tried, to keep a foot in that normal world, the world which did not revolve around my cancer, but it was hard. My diary of this time is full of this person and that person coming to visit me at home – my family, friends. There are even appointments for facials. There are weekends in Shropshire. Life carried on. But only after a fashion, in a surface way.

My life gradually became ruled by hospital appointments, by my reactions to the drugs I was given and my energy levels. My hair started to fall out, more of which later, and each time I thought I'd got a handle on my physical state, it seemed to change. I hadn't been back to work – my chemo started 20 days after my mastectomy, just when I probably would have gone back – and I seemed to spend my days cancelling and rearranging visitors and appointments. There were days when I felt okay, but I was never sure when they would be, and even on good days I was often tired and had to rest in the afternoon. So many other days drifted by in a fog of nausea, and when the nausea faded, I was so constipated by the anti-emetics I had taken that I had to take drugs for that, and became paranoid that I would explode if I went out. It happened to me once in

Tom's, the trendy café in Notting Hill, where I had dragged myself to meet a friend, desperate to get out of the house, exercise my body a little. How long can you stay in a loo when it's the only one in the whole café? And how do you explain your prolonged absence to your companion? It was just too much information again.

My illness gradually took up so much of my time that I could no longer keep it in what I thought of as its place, control it. I felt myself *becoming my illness*, the sum of my symptoms. I was not me, the me I knew. I became what I had been all along, but had not fully accepted – someone with cancer. That, I realised, is why chemo is the endgame, is so feared. There's no pretending any more when you have chemo, and it had turned me into someone who was not only not up to working, but not up to running her home or looking after her children. It had turned me into a burden. It was terrifying. One of the abiding memories of this time for me is of feeling trapped, trapped in bed, trapped on the sofa, the hours ticking slowly by and nothing, absolutely nothing happening, and being completely unable to make anything happen, sometimes unable to even make myself a cup of tea. I felt infantilised. *Torture*. When I recently saw Mike Nichols' film, *Angels in America*, about AIDS in America in the Eighties, I was struck by how much I identified with the rage and humiliation the men felt at the way illness took away their independence, their ability to lead a normal life, their self-respect.

I was terrified by what I saw at the hospital. On one of my visits to the chemo suite, I was asked to go with another patient, to meet her at the lift. She, apparently, was also having problems being cannulated. When I saw her, I was horrified.

She was skeletal, bald, hunched. She wasn't that much older than me. She was also friendly. She chatted away. But I could hardly speak. I wanted to run away. *This was not going to be me, I thought*. But I also knew that it might well be me, maybe not right now but maybe later.

I went to a relaxation class organised by the oncology department. I was the youngest by about 20 years. When I sat down, an elderly woman asked me what I 'had'. Breast cancer, I said. Oh, she said. I had that eight years ago. Now I've got it in me tubes. *Eight years ago? Would I never be free?*

The clinic where I waited to see Professor Coombes, with its plastic chairs and ancient magazines, was discouraging. I was flanked by bad wigs, lopsided chests, faces bloated by steroids, heads with lightning bolts etched on their skulls. I watched the shufflers who took an eternity to reach the reception desk, the wild-eyed emergencies who crashed through the door and went straight into one of the doctor's rooms; no signing in for them, no time. I listened to the wheezers. *These were my people now.*

My fortieth birthday fell on the Sunday before one of the last chemo sessions. We had spent the weekend at the cottage and it was a sunny day. I can't remember much about it except that it wasn't how I'd imagined it would be. I didn't give a damn about turning 40 as such. I've never been able to understand why people worry about their age, lie about their age. I know women, more and more it would seem, who are forever 39, who were, when we first met, older than me, but are now younger, and I have a friend who will not tell me how old she is at all. It seems an odd way of carrying on. So I wasn't vexed in the way that women are supposed to be about turning 40. In some ways, I'd been looking forward to it. Simon had loved being 40, found it liberating. I had thought I might celebrate, do something special to mark the occasion. But now I was wondering whether I would ever make 41 and a special day for me now was an ordinary day, a day when I didn't feel sick. That was the kind of knees-up I dreamed of. No champagne, no dancing, just a day at home with Simon and the children when I wasn't in bed all day, maybe just for a rest in the afternoon.

And I've felt like that about birthdays ever since, not in some drippy, live-for-the-moment way, but birthdays now always remind me that, during that summer, an ordinary day was a blessing. I am also glad to watch myself grow older. As I write this, I am 46. I am proud to say I'm 46, a little boastful perhaps. I'm thrilled to see lines round my eyes, grey hairs. When I hear friends who are older talking about what it's like to be 50, I'm filled with longing. Some are complaining about those lines, their changing bodies, that their lives have stalled. Some are joyful, full of plans. I want to be able to discuss these things, to see which camp I fall into. Back then, on my fortieth birthday though, my greatest ambition was to have one ordinary day.

When I finished my course of outpatients chemo, I thought, hoped maybe, that I might have more ordinary days. I also thought I would feel relieved. It wasn't like that though. I had the stem cell transplant to think about. The trouble is, though, that as soon as I started trying to think about it, I realised I couldn't. My brain refused to cooperate. It was September. I had a vague admission date for the Hammersmith for mid-October, vague because I had to wait for a bed. No more private wards for me. Stem cell transplants were carried out on one particular specialist ward geared up for keeping patients in the semi-isolation that was necessary to protect impaired immune systems, and that was that.

One of the problems I had with the treatment was that nobody, apart from a few doctors, had ever heard of it. From the moment I had discovered the lump in my breast, I had felt myself being dragged into another world and that feeling of otherness had increased with each step of my treatment. But what had helped keep me tentatively in the normal world was language. The basic words – cancer, surgery and chemotherapy – had some resonance with other people. Not always the right or the most helpful resonance, but at least some resonance. The words stem cell transplant did not and I found it hard to enlighten them because I couldn't get to grips with it myself. It was a new-ish technique. Professor Coombes told me that people felt quite ill during the treatment, often had stomach problems. The hospital gave me a photocopy of a patient's description of it. CancerBACUP – the charity which, alongside its telephone helpline, produces booklets and leaflets on all aspects of cancer and its treatment – had, at the time, little to say about it. *Dr Susan Love's Breast Book*, the breast cancer bible which, in those pre-Amazon.com days, Anna had lugged back from America for me, seemed sceptical about its benefits. The *New Yorker* article which described it as the killing cure was published much later. This lack of information, of being at the frontiers of medicine, made me feel vulnerable, out of control, and I hated it.

In my terror, I fixated on what would happen to the children while I was hospitalised, how to minimise their trauma, something I thought I could exercise some control over. I had been told by Professor Coombes that there was a counsellor attached to the oncology unit who I might want to talk to if I had any worries about the treatment, so I took my concerns about the children to her. I had not, up to this point, considered seeing a counsellor. In my confusion, I had concluded that my fears were so obvious, so lacking in mystery, that they didn't need unravelling, deconstructing. I was wrong, but that's how I felt at the time. I did, however, feel comfortable asking for advice on how to manage the stem cell transplant. The counsellor, a neat, pretty woman, had a tiny room in the radiotherapy department. It was precisely furnished with two nasty pastel sofas and a little table on which sat a box of pastel tissues.

'Why do you think your children shouldn't see you?' she said.

'It will be too traumatic for them.'

'Why?'

Wasn't it obvious, I thought. This woman is useless. Then, much to my surprise, I started crying.

'I'm so frightened,' I said.

I now know that she was a cognitive therapist and she did help me through this period in a magnificently practical way. She asked me to visualise myself in the hospital. What would I be wearing? What would I be doing? What would the room be like? Who would be around me? This made it more manageable, less frightening. She also questioned my theory that the children would be traumatised if they came to visit me. For this insight, I shall be forever grateful. She said that she thought they might be more traumatised not knowing where I was, imagining where I was, and that, in her experience, many children had seen hospital programmes on TV and, when visiting hospitals, were more interested in the equipment than anything else. I realised that what I had been worried about was how *I* would feel, seeing my children see me. I had got stuck on the detail again because I could not bear to think about the bigger picture, the seriousness of my situation, the awfulness of it. It's not that my concerns about the children were ridiculous – they were perfectly natural – but I was using these concerns as a smokescreen for my own fears. It's not to say, either, that Lucian and Cosima were not traumatised by my having cancer, just that they were not particularly bothered by the hi-tech hospital unit. When they did visit me, they were amazed by the TV in my room, the bed which went up and down, my cards, the room down the corridor where there was a kettle and microwave. They reacted much as they had when they had visited me in hospital before, when I was, in my mind, less compromised as a functioning mother. They showed scant interest in the complicated drip stand with its hanging bags to which I was attached and how appalling I felt I looked.

The other suggestion the counsellor made was that I did not have to organise every last second of my family's life during my hospital stay. I had been trying to do this with lists and plans. It was another way of pretending that I had control over my situation, but it was also a genuine worry. I was and am the organiser in our family. Simon has always done most of the cooking and food shopping, but I have always held that particular bigger picture in my head, organising the children, Kerry, Siony, the house, school, our finances, everything from clean sheets to nit remedies and new shoes. I would be out of action for at least a month. What would happen to my little family without me? I became obsessed with this, and behind this question always lurked the other question. *What would happen to my little family if I died?* My cancer was gradually and inexorably taking me away from my family, my absences becoming ever longer, and the stem cell treatment was starting to feel like a practice run for my permanent absence.

So when the counsellor said they would cope, and said it confidently, I couldn't believe her, wouldn't believe her, because, if I did, I felt I was somehow saying it was okay for me to die. And when she asked me other questions about how I felt about my cancer, I fobbed her off. I couldn't listen to her because I couldn't bear to hear her taking the situation so seriously. She told me a story about a woman who, on her deathbed, was agonising about leaving her children in the care of their father from whom she was estranged and did not trust. I don't have those sort of worries, I said. And I didn't, at least not in the most superficial of ways. I trusted Simon but I could not bring myself to think about such a scenario. It was beyond me.

It was easy, too, to find no time to stand and stare. There was the endless prepping, for a start. I had my heart tested – saw it pumping away on a screen and listened to its whoosh-whoosh. I had my lungs tested. I had a guided tour of the unit where I would be treated, with its single rooms, ensuite bathrooms and TVs. I signed a form to say that I understood I could die during treatment. I also had to say that I understood why I could die – I might come down with an untreatable infection during the period after the high-dose chemo when my immune system would be, well, non-functioning – and I laughed along with the doctor when he told me that they hadn't lost anyone yet. I had my kidneys tested – carrying around a large plastic container into which I had to pee for 24 hours. I took it out clothes shopping with me, hiding it in a big handbag. In fact, I seemed to spend almost as much time shopping for clothes as I did having tests.

I bought a skirt and shirt from Issey Miyake. I bought a cardigan from Voyage. Expensive stuff. Pretty stuff. My mother thought the cardigan was a bedjacket. I didn't need these clothes. They were the kind of things I'd often thought about buying – one day, maybe, when I won the lottery – but hadn't. I had mortgages, nannies and nurseries to pay for. Expensive clothes were low down on my list of priorities, occasional purchases. Now I wasn't sure what my priorities were and bought lots. And wore them – to work where I had returned briefly, on the school run, recklessly over-dressed.

The Issey Miyake outfit also had another significance for me. I had always admired his clothes. They are works of art, made from strange crushed and pleated fabrics which curve softly round the body. They are inspired by the swaddled, bandaged bodies of the victims of Hiroshima. But like most such high-concept clothes, they are nigh on unwearable, can look ridiculous, unless you are very striking or work in an art gallery – or are old. Somehow they look fabulous on older women. And those thoughts of bandages and old age drove me into the shop. I felt like being swaddled, perhaps in some ways I felt like I had been in a nuclear attack myself, and I no longer had any faith in being old so, I thought, I'd better have my Issey Miyake moment now. It cheered me up, as did the Voyage cardigan. During this period, I also became obsessed with bath and body lotions, scented, soothing oils and lotions. I was desperate for an antidote to the knives and needles and poisons to which my body had been subjected. I was also, I think, prepping myself in a different way from the doctors. With the worst to come, I needed to bank some gentleness, some self-indulgence to get me through.

During this period, I also had an extraordinary stroke of luck. My friend Vinny, who I had not seen for a long time, appeared out of nowhere, on a white charger. She had been working in Paris and tracked me down through another friend, Gill, and asked me if I would like to meet her friend Francine who had had the same treatment. I did. *Of course I did*.

I went to see Francine for lunch. She seemed reticent, spoke carefully, which I put down to being post-treatment and not wanting to go back over old ground. Now, I suspect, she didn't want to frighten me too much. I was, I can remember, concerned about how I would pass the time for a whole month in hospital. What could you do when you were in semi-isolation? I had been told that I could have visitors but that it would be better if the number was limited – and that, of course, nobody with a cold or other infection should visit me, which was alarming given that I would be hospitalised late autumn, the beginning of the cold season. More alarming though was the idea I had that I would be bored. I saw endless empty hours to fill. How did you entertain yourself, I asked Francine. She said she had taken a lot of stuff into hospital with her, but hadn't really felt up to doing much. She described how she had tried to do some yoga on the floor, but then couldn't get herself back into bed. We laughed. She was telling me what it was like, but I wasn't ready to hear what she was saying.

When I look back, my state of mind reminds me of myself before I had Lucian, a state of wilful ignorance. I had planned to stop work two weeks before my due date and then take three months' maternity leave. This seemed like an eternity to me. The longest holiday I'd ever had was three weeks. I bought a new Filofax to reorganise my address book. I bought a tapestry. *A tapestry?* I stockpiled books to read. I planned three trips, one just four weeks after my due date. I had friends with children, I had friends who, apparently – I have to believe them because they later told me so – I had listened to sympathetically when they told me their tales of sleepless nights and near-constant state of panic when their first child was born. But somehow I could not imagine how different my life would be with a baby. I could not imagine being at home, not working, and yet having no free time. I could not imagine a life where a Filofax and tapestry could languish untouched in their carrier bags, where a few simple trips, to Lyme Regis, to Wales and to France, would prove a challenge too far and that, back in London, I would consider getting dressed by lunchtime a significant achievement.

And now I could not imagine what this stem cell transplant would be like. So I ignored the warning signals Francine sent me and organised a laptop, a mobile phone – not ubiquitous then – books, magazines, tapes, a radio, videos.

I had been told that I would get a call from the Hammersmith as soon as a bed came free. It could be earlier or later than the date I had been given (a Sunday), so I should be prepared for either. The treatment was unpredictable, the hospital said. Sometimes people stayed in longer than anticipated or suddenly rallied. The Saturday before my date I was told that they were on schedule, but that I would be rung again on the Sunday afternoon to confirm. My parents were coming to lunch. My mother had offered to stay and act as Simon's back-up for the children in case he needed to be with me at the hospital in the evening. We had fish pie. I wanted something filling, nutritious. It felt like my last supper. Then, at around 2pm, the ward rang saying I should report at 4pm.

We went for a walk, to Brompton Cemetery. This was not as bizarre as it sounds. The cemetery is beautiful, Victorian, huge, and five minutes from the flat. It is where we go for walks, safe bike rides. It is full of people walking, feeding the squirrels and, in the summer, sitting in the sun. Back then, it was also full of gay men cruising. There seem to be not so many now. There was no morbid significance to our choice of venue and my only memory of the walk is that, on the way to the cemetery, as we walked past the number 14 bus stop in the Fulham Road, I started crying and I tried to walk behind the children, so that they wouldn't see my tears. They were tears of fear, of loneliness, despite being surrounded by people who loved me. In the summer, when I had broken down in front of my parents, sobbing about how frightened I was, my mother had said that I should try to remember that I wasn't alone. And I wasn't, in that I had the most incredible support. And I was, in that I often felt existentially alone. This was one of those times.

I remember that it was a sunny day, one of those autumnal high-pressure days, the sky bright blue and spotless, my favourite kind of weather. Or it was. Back then, I was never a fan of summer. It was fine in the countryside, I thought, but London just stank in the heat. It was noisy and filthy. The winter? Not so fine in the countryside – hard work – but in London, I felt it drifted by in a blur, everyone staying inside, dashing from home to school, work, blanking out the weather as much as possible. Spring and autumn were, to me, the best seasons in the city, the temperature right for walking, looking up instead of down, and admiring the architecture. High-pressure days also reminded me of my first morning in New York and, walking out of the Chelsea Hotel looking for Fifth Avenue, suddenly finding myself dazzled by the buildings glinting in the light, all at once realising what the city was all about.

But that October day in 1997 destroyed that feeling of exhilaration for me for many years and it took many years to unravel another sinister side-effect. Even now, every autumn I start to feel anxious. I feel confused. Then, one seemingly random day, I look up at the sky and I realise why I feel anxious: I am remembering that day, but my subconscious has remembered it before my conscious mind. The weather is the trigger. In retrospect, it is an obvious pattern, but for many years it was like looking at one of those children's puzzles where, within a mass of squiggles and dots, hides a picture of a clown, a rabbit. Before you see it, you cannot see it at all, but once you have seen it, you cannot imagine why you could not see it.

At the hospital, I was, at first, parked in a general cancer ward. I sat on the bed, fully clothed, feeling self-conscious. There were five other people in the ward. They didn't look great. I may have been a bit pale and thin, but compared to everyone else I radiated health. I was also the youngest by at least 10 years. A student nurse came to see me. She said she wanted to ask me a few questions. It turned out that she wanted my entire medical history. At first, I was polite, but as she stumbled along – sorry, did you say it was your left or your right breast? – I became gradually angrier and then I said I couldn't carry on. This is ridiculous, I said. I'm being admitted for a serious procedure and you're asking me what's wrong with me. Surely you have a file on me. I then asked if I could be moved up to the private wing to wait. *Little Miss Snooty*. I couldn't, so we sat and waited. For hours.

I was taken off to have a Hickman line put in, a version of the central line which I had had for the stem cell harvest. It was just as humiliating second time round and, back on the ward, I cried again. In the next bed was a woman with lung cancer. She was slumped in a chair which was where she was going to sleep. She couldn't lie down. She was wheezing, uncomfortable. It was frightening. Opposite was a woman in her sixties. She'd been given the wrong sandwich for supper and sat, miserable and hungry, staring into space.

Later that night, I was taken up to my room on the specialist ward. It was a gloomy little room, with a tiny window looking on to a brick wall. They said I would be moved to one of the rooms nearer the nurses' station when it came free; they were bigger, sunnier, they said cheerfully. Nothing would be happening that night though. I asked if I could go home. Amazingly, they said yes, as long as I reported back first thing.

At home, Simon made pasta. I had a glass or two of red

wine. It might as well have been heroin, I was on such a high. I slept soundly that night, and when I went back to the hospital the next day, I was calmer. The following day, I moved into the bigger room.

It is hard now to believe that I was only in hospital for a month. I do not have absolute recall of this period. I just have snapshots in my mind. Yet, afterwards, I suffered from a form of post-traumatic stress in that I could not process the experience, absorb it. It was too unusual an experience, so outside of my normal terms of reference, beyond my linguistic ability. I could not explain it to myself or other people. The snapshots, of course, are not happy snaps. They are more like the kind of pictures the police take after some gruesome incident.

In practical terms, I was given the high-dose chemotherapy through the Hickman line for around four days, continuously. By my bed was the drip stand. The bags of chemicals were hung on this and attached to the dangling ports on my line. The stand was plugged into a socket by the bed and the chemicals dripped through automatically. It bleeped if there were problems. When I went to the bathroom, I had to unplug the stand and wheel it in with me. The only time I was allowed to be disconnected was when I had a bath. As soon as the chemo started, I started throwing up. It was quite dramatic and coincided with a surprise visit from one of the writers at the newspaper. She was in the middle of telling me about her contract negotiations with my boss when suddenly I vomited, almost but not quite projectilely. She gamely tried to continue with her story and then, luckily, my sister Julie arrived and gently ushered her out. It was a glimpse of how things would be throughout this period. I craved companionship, people who were rooting for me, but I was unable to cope with visits – or even phone calls – from anyone who needed me to respond to them. Not that they made me throw up. I simply had no energy to play any kind of hostess.

In fact, the vomiting was short-lived. I was given anti-emetics intravenously and, from then on, I just felt nauseous. I developed diarrhoea. I couldn't eat or drink. The chemo, I was told, had burned my gut.

After the chemo, I was given back my white blood cells, again through the Hickman line. That was the easy bit of the treatment over. I was now, the doctors told me, on Day One. My immune system had been destroyed and I had to wait for it to rise from the dead, for the white blood cells to proliferate, for the stem cells or mother cells to go forth and multiply. This, I was told, would take about 10 days. During that period, I would be prone to infection so would be given antibiotics, again intravenously. My temperature would be taken frequently as a rise would indicate an infection. The infections they were worried about were internal, the infections we unknowingly fight off daily. My blood would be taken frequently, too, to ascertain any problems. I would be given various blood products. I would also be given chest X-rays, in bed.

Time seemed to stand still during those ten days. I lay on my bed, more or less flat. The view out of the window was a patch of grey sky and a pylon. I did not have the energy to sit up and I didn't much care. I did not read. I did not listen to the radio. I did not listen to tapes. In the evening, I watched TV. Sometimes in the day, I watched videos. I liked comedy shows best – *Ab Fab* and *Father Ted*. I tried to watch the film *Trainspotting*, which I had missed when it came out, but zoned out after the lavatory scene. My sisters came to visit. In the mornings, my mother, father or Anna came to sit with me. Simon was there most afternoons and every evening until I fell asleep, when the sleeping pill I insisted on kicked in. It was only later that I could see how complicated this must have been to arrange and how driven Simon had been to help me feel less alone. Even at the time, though, I was aware of how hard it was for visitors to be with me. Simon, in particular, was heroic. A fidget by nature, he endured hours of enforced inactivity with charming grace. I was not good company. The hours, the days drifted by. I felt like a note left in a pocket and put in the wash, soft, worn, faded, unreadable, useless.

I tried to keep still – the nausea lingered. I tried to lengthen the gap between the bouts of diarrhoea. I had to write down every sip of liquid I drank – pitiful. I also had to pee into a jug and measure the urine before flushing it down the loo. Sometimes I felt so weak that I couldn't walk the few yards to the bathroom and peed into the jug as I crouched by the bed. Once, in the night, I was so confused that I peed all over the bed.

I tried to eat, but couldn't. I was only allowed cooked food or individually wrapped boxes of cereal or biscuits because of the risk of contamination. I nibbled at bourbons. I ordered a baked potato, every day, from the appalling menu. My visitor would mush it up for me and I would push it round the plate until it was stone cold. Some days, I was brought the wrong food and, once, a potato so hard that it couldn't be mashed, only sliced. The food, apparently, was prepared at Wormwood Scrubs prison which lurked behind the huge fences at the back of the hospital.

At one point I was put on a drip because I was losing too much weight and was given a selection of disgusting slimy build-up drinks. Most were lime flavour.

The high point of my day was my bath, which I had around 3pm. Simon helped me in and out. I had to be careful with the Hickman line. He washed my hair which was getting thinner and thinner. I slapped on an expensive body lotion and face cream, and changed my nightdress. I collect vintage white cotton and linen nightdresses and the nurses found them amusing with their billows and lace. Each day I sent home one or two with Simon and they came back washed and ironed by Kerry.

I had been warned that I might develop mouth ulcers, so I brushed my teeth carefully and rinsed my mouth with a special wash. The ulcers never appeared. I developed a pain in my stomach though and it was suggested that I have an X-ray. This one couldn't be done in my bed so I would have to go to the X-ray unit at the other end of the hospital. A wheelchair was brought into the room. A mask was put on my face to reduce the possibility of infection. I shrugged on my dressing gown and was helped into the wheelchair. I was pushed, quickly, through the corridors to the X-ray department. This was the first time I had been outside my room in over two weeks. People stared at me. I was pale, hunched. Half my hair was missing and what was left was in a state, tufty. I felt like a freak. When I got to the department, I was wheeled straight in. No waiting for me. I was asked by the technician, who kept his distance from me, to climb on to the bench in the middle of the room. I wasn't sure I could. I lurched around unsteadily before finally making it. As soon as the X-ray had been taken, I shakily rolled myself off and was wheeled back to the ward.

Shortly after, I decided to have my head shaved. I gave up pretending I was me, the me that was. Which was good because that was really what was required of me, to become a non-person, to view my body objectively. The goal, during those two weeks when my body was at ground zero, was basic survival, and until that had been achieved, everything else, my feelings, my future, was on hold. I was not a mother, a partner, a daughter, a journalist. I was a body. Not surprisingly, I resisted this way of looking at my life. It seemed so recently that I had thought basic survival was the lowest of goals. How could it, so suddenly, have become the highest?

Much later, when I took a psychology course, I learned about Maslow's hierarchy of needs, the list of requirements which need to be fulfilled in our lives before we can self-actualise, become truly fulfilled. It is usually illustrated as a triangle, with food, shelter, etc. at the wide bottom of the triangle, and self-actualisation as the pinnacle, the tip. One of the most basic needs, a serious chunk of the triangle, is safety. I was not safe. I was in great danger. I had plummeted from near the top of the triangle to the bottom in a matter of months. It would take much longer to climb back up.

In my worst moments, I thought that if I reached a point where there was no hope of getting better, no hope of my immune system recovering, where I would only get worse, then I would want to die, be put to sleep, killed, I suppose. Basic survival was not enough. It wasn't living. I understood, in a different way, the arguments for euthanasia. One night, I had a terrifying dream. I was on a trolley in a side corridor, a place which seemed dark, untidy, unsafe. I was surrounded by jeering doctors. They were trying to smother me in an offhand kind of way and I couldn't move. I woke up sweating and frightened. The images were a jumble of my worst experiences, their significance horribly clear. My life was in jeopardy, death was stalking me.

In my better moments, I watched hours of *Ab Fab* videos while I sipped from a carton of build-up drink.

The nurses helped. They were the best that I have ever encountered, intelligent, kind. They were specialists, technical wizards, used to dealing with extremes. They chatted as they administered their poisons, the lifesavers. They told me about their shifts, their children, their childcare. I wanted them to earn a million pounds a week and felt guilty at the money I earned doing nothing for anyone. They all seemed to be called Kate, which I liked.

Every now and then, a consultant appeared. He was pompous, surrounded by nervous students and junior doctors. He stood at the end of my bed and asked me how I was, told me he knew someone on the board of the company I worked for. He used the phrase 'gippy tummy', barked at his nervous acolytes and swept out again. Not surprisingly, I never developed any relationship with him, or the other doctors in charge of my treatment at the Hammersmith, which is strange when I think how important, how dangerous, it was. I continued to think of Professor Coombes as my guardian angel.

As the day approached when my immune system was supposed to normalise, I was given GCSF again, to speed things along. I was given a hot water bottle for the bone pain and hid under the sheets like a child, trying to visualise the pain ebbing away and the white blood cells flooding my body. And then a couple of days later it happened. I felt better. I no longer felt as sick. I could nibble at food. I could – and wanted to – sit up. And then I wanted to leave the hospital as soon as possible. The hospital wanted me to go soon, too, but I had to wait for my blood levels to stabilise. I was encouraged to leave my room for short periods, to practise walking. Finally I was given a release date but was told that, up until the last minute, it was subject to change.

On the day, Simon and my mother came together to get me. I was given some more tests and then told, yes, I could go. I put on a big furry hat and a coat. I walked very slowly, holding on to Simon, to the lift and out to the car park. I felt like someone who had been blind and had regained their sight. Everything seemed bright, technicolor. There was so much to look at and it seemed so noisy. We stopped for petrol and I drank in the bustle, the normality of it all. When I got home, I crawled up the flights of stairs to the flat and flopped on to the sofa, overwhelmed by the colours and textures, the stuff, my stuff. I was, in my own very modest way, Nelson Mandela on that long walk to freedom.

4

Imitation Of Life

Now, whenever I think about my cancer treatment, I think of that stem cell transplant as the grand finale. There was more — five weeks of daily radiotherapy and five years of taking tamoxifen, the breast cancer drug, every day — but they are, to me, a mere postscript. Both were irritating, but as nothing compared with that month in the hospital.

The medical follow-up was alarmingly low-key after four weeks of round-the-clock intensive care. I felt confused as to how best I should look after myself. Should I rest? Should I push myself? Should I expect any after-effects? I had no idea. I had a few drugs to take, but not many and not for long. I had to go back for a check-up, but only one. In the end, it was Lucian and Cosima who forced the pace of my recovery, for which I am grateful. Without their demands, their hungriness for normal family life to resume, I may have been tempted to act the southern belle. The first night back, they asked me to put them to bed and, amazingly, I did. I staggered up the stairs to read them a story, lying down on the floor between their beds because I didn't have the energy to sit up. It was the right thing for me to do, fast-forwarding my physical confidence. My mother stayed over that night and sat with me the next day while Simon went to work, in case I felt bad. I did suddenly feel nauseous again and had to ring the hospital to ask if I should take some of my old anti-emetic medication. But soon after, I rallied and I quickly got into a routine of getting up in the morning with everyone else and having a nap in the afternoon so that I could go to bed at a normal time, too.

I gradually got stronger and, apart from one terrifying incident when I passed an enormous blood clot – apparently, a phantom period, the result of the drugs I had been taking – the most noticeable side-effect of the treatment was on my appetite. After weeks of eating almost nothing, I was now ravenous. But my stomach seemed to have shrunk and I felt so frail that I had to gradually increase the amount and variety of foods I ate. Simon, a wonderful cook, patiently prepared small portions of mashed potato, little dishes of pasta, toddler food. I didn't have the energy to sit at the table, and ate on the sofa, feet up, with a tray. I couldn't get enough calories with my mini breakfasts, lunches and suppers, so I ate every couple of hours, even through the night. When I went up to bed, I took a glass of Coke with me and a packet of digestive biscuits, my old standbys for morning sickness, which I would snack on at regular intervals,

Not very healthy, you probably think. But there's an awful lot of rubbish talked about cancer and diet. Up until my diagnosis I had always had a healthy diet: grilled this, grilled that, lots of vegetables, rarely puddings. I drank, but only red wine and not so much. I took supplements on and off.

There is, I know, much evidence that some cancers are linked to diet. But I have never seen any convincing evidence that diet

has any effect once cancer has developed. There are famous cancer diets – notably the Gerson and Bristol Cancer Centre regimes, both of which require enormous commitment. The two people I have come across who followed the Gerson diet both had assistants to help them prepare their food. I was told about these diets many times by friends and acquaintances and, although my instinct was to steer clear of them, I did ask Dr Charles Lowdell, the consultant who oversaw my radiotherapy, about them. I was curious because no medical person had ever asked me about my diet. His response took me by surprise, at first.

'I have a lot of patients on these diets,' he said. 'They seem to find them helpful.'

'Oh. So you think I should go on one of these diets?'

'Do you want to?'

'No.'

'Well, don't then.'

'But if it would help . . .'

'I said my patients find them helpful. I, personally, have never seen these diets have any effect on outcome.'

Outcome, that little word that stands in for survival.

'I don't think I'll bother then.'

'It's up to you, but it's really about how you want to spend your time now. Perhaps grating carrots is not how you want to spend it.'

Many years later, a nutritionist who came to talk at Gilda's Club, the cancer support charity where I was working, summed up the dilemma in a different way. She said that when you ride a motorbike, you wear a crash helmet. When you have a motorbike accident and get taken to casualty, the doctors don't prescribe a crash helmet for your injuries. Nutrition, she said, should be seen as the crash helmet, cancer, the accident. What counted for most cancer patients in the treatment phase, she said, was calories.

And that's what I was concentrating on with my Coke and biscuits at night – I could also consume them quickly and quietly in the dark without disturbing Simon. I would never recommend that anyone live on Coke and biscuits, but when you are ill, particularly when you are feeling nauseous or losing too much weight, you don't need people bugging you about your diet. You need food that you find palatable and that gives you calories. I had cream and sugar with everything. I found tea with sugar and some squares of chocolate a most acceptable snack. Greek yogurt with honey was good, too. For a while. Because the other point about this topsy-turvy way of eating was that it was, for me, short term. As my stomach went back to normal – well, as normal as it was ever going to be – I went back to regular meals and normal food again. Other people die. And who wants to spend their last months denying themselves doughnuts if that's what they really fancy and can stomach.

Simon came into his own – yet again – over the food issue. He has never had any truck with fad diets. He is adamant, however, that people should eat proper food, as opposed to convenience food, and eat a little of everything. There are no bad foods in his eyes. He also believes that food should be enjoyed, and an important part of our life together as a couple – and, later, as a family once the children started eating regular food – is eating together. Even during the years when I worked long hours, we tried to eat together, and colleagues were often baffled by the great lengths I would go to in order to get home for a late supper with Simon rather than take things slowly then drift off to the pub with them. And once I was nearing the end of my treatment, I felt Simon was as motivated as I was – and sometimes more so when I balked at larger portions – to build up my stamina and appetite.

By the time Christmas approached, I was on the home stretch. I just about managed to do the Christmas present shopping and we held our usual family fish pie and champagne get-together at the flat, then I tried to settle into a normal diet. I think I ate more though and, if I fancied something fattening, I ate it. But apart from that I changed my diet very little. For a while, we bought organic wine and milk, and I decided that I would take the Bristol Cancer Centre's recommended list of supplements once my radiotherapy was over – and did, for a couple of years. Now, if I feel I need nutritional advice, I look at one of Jane Clarke's books. They are full of common sense.

In the middle of December, I went to see Professor Coombes. He gave me my prescription for tamoxifen, the hormonal treatment I had puzzled over in my consultations with Mr Sinnett, which works on the oestrogen in the body and was considered helpful to me as my tumour was oestrogen-positive. I asked a few questions about the side-effects I'd heard about – weight gain, hot flushes – but it was a pretty pointless exercise. I was going to take the stuff whatever he said. Simon asked, only half-joking, if I would grow a moustache, develop a deep voice, turn into a man in other words. Professor Coombes said he'd never seen that happen. I was then sent along to see Dr Lowdell about my radiotherapy.

He talked me through the protocol – the five days a week for five weeks, with check-ups once a week – and then did an extraordinary thing. He asked me and Simon how we were coping. We were so taken aback, so used to dealing with the detail by then, that we didn't know what to say. His enquiry was to have a profound effect on me.

I arranged to have my radiotherapy at the Cromwell as it was nearer home and went along just before Christmas with Simon and the children to be prepped. I didn't really want to take the children, but school was out and Kerry was away, and I didn't want to go alone. The radiotherapy unit is in the basement of the hospital, and the waiting room is cosy with armchairs and a TV. I was taken into a large room, asked to lie on a trolley and lights like laser beams were shone on to my body as the technicians worked out exactly where I would be blasted. My body was then marked with two indelible dots – which, briefly, made me think of Auschwitz again – which would be used as locator marks. I still have them. I was told that, throughout the treatment, I couldn't wash the area – my breast and armpit – or use deodorant. I was given a tube of aloe vera lotion to keep the skin supple. In the end, I cheated a bit and splashed the area with water. But I was lucky – it was winter, not summer when I would have been mortified at not using a deodorant.

My treatment was to start in January and I was asked, this being a private hospital, what time I would like to attend each day. I chose 9.10am. I had decided that I could manage this part of the treatment on my own and I thought that I could drop Lucian off at school, then go straight on to the hospital. Afterwards, I could pop into Sainsbury's next door before going home. My days were relatively free to recover and rest. This convenience factor was very pleasing to me and gave me back a much-missed sense of being in control of my life, my time.

Radiotherapy takes minutes. It doesn't hurt. I had no side-effects except, for a while, a faint discoloration of my breast — it's different if you have radiotherapy on or near your stomach, bowel or brain when you can feel quite sick. It wasn't frightening — again, different if you have radiotherapy on your head when you have to wear a specially made mask which makes you look like R2D2. It is odd though.

You walk into an enormous room and lie on a bench in the middle of the room. Your body is arranged by the technicians — I had to lie in a strange, Egon Schiele position with my arm bent round my head and my armpit bared. The technicians then leave the room, at speed. You are told to lie completely still and then it happens, the radiotherapy. You feel absolutely nothing, yet you know that the technicians don't want to be anywhere near you, that certain amounts of radiation can treat cancer, more can cause it. After a couple of minutes, a voice comes over the intercom: time to go home.

Some people get tired during radiotherapy, their fatigue increased by the travelling to the hospital every day, the emotional trauma. It took me five minutes to walk to the hospital from Lucian's school, 15 minutes to walk home. For me, it was a piece of cake compared with the stem cell transplant. I had a few hiccups. I got pains in my calves, once so bad that I collapsed in the street. I was scanned. Nothing. I got flu — the shivering, can't-get-out-of-bed kind — as did Simon. It was a Sunday and my parents had to come up for the day to look after the children.

The next day I went for my radiotherapy, dragging myself along the street, hunched and sweating in the freezing cold. I shouldn't miss it, the hospital said.

These things were just hiccups though, nothing more. Overall, my wellbeing and strength were more stable than they had been for months. But I wasn't happy. I hadn't, of course, been happy for months, but I had been occupied. Now that my treatment was demanding less of me physically and psychologically, and my schedule was becoming more predictable and manageable, I was starting to have the time and mental energy to look beyond the immediate. I couldn't think clearly though – a fog would descend whenever I tried to think about my situation. I yo-yoed between denial and tentative acknowledgment of my predicament. It was a miserable experience.

I was, according to Simon, very quiet during this period, but I was unaware of this. My mind was racing. Nowhere. Thoughts would go round and round and round, but I never came to any conclusions because I couldn't work out what I was debating. The nub of the thing eluded me, but I was convinced that if I tried hard enough I would be able to work out what it was and that once I knew what the problem was, I would be able to solve it. I exhausted myself. If you had seen me then, I would have looked idle, resting up. But in my head I was running a marathon, in sand. I hadn't a clue about the route or where the finishing line was.

I felt unhappy in a different way from when I was diagnosed and during my treatment. There had been an inevitability about my unhappiness before and most of the time I felt merely flat, numb, with occasional breakouts of rudeness and rage. One morning at the cottage, soon after my diagnosis, I came downstairs into the empty kitchen and was shocked to find myself wanting to smash everything in sight. I stood, stock still, imagining doing this, then walked out into the garden to cool down. In fact, the cottage often unearthed powerful emotions in me. Back then, we spent most weekends there and Saturday evening was a quiet time for Simon and me together without the distraction of television or work to catch up on, and I would frequently start weeping during dinner and find it hard to stop. As we set off back to London on Sunday evening, I would often weep once more, convinced that I would never see the cottage again. I don't think this had anything to do with the fact that I had discovered the lump while there, more that it was a place which represented so much to me. It was an achievement, a place of refuge where we were together as a family, somewhere I had grown to love and often longed to be when I was in London.

This longing had little to do with playing farms, Marie Antoinette-style, and everything to do with feeling free, off-piste. The cottage was also the repository for so many memories of family life, those little anecdotes that mean nothing to anybody else and everything to me, Simon and the children. Being snowed in, foxes chasing rabbits, a four-year-old Lucian herding cows out of the garden, baby Cosima squashed in the carrycot at night like a dolly in a box, Simon's first fabulous crop of potatoes, my growing collection of old baskets and quilts, days spent gardening, cooking, reading by the fire, walking in the woods, visits from family and friends. We all have our stories about holidays there. Such small things, but they added up to what I felt was the real texture of my life, what I was in danger of losing, partly or wholly. As a result, the cottage somehow had the ability to unhinge me, the dark side of its ability to make me happy.

It did this at the most unlikely moments. It happened once on the way back from a walk in the woods. The house was below us, halfway down the hill, invisible tethers keeping it from the freedom of the fields and woodland beyond. The descent to the house was steep, too steep. I tried to negotiate it with dignity, but the children abandoned themselves to the sensation of speed, shrieking with masochistic glee. Simon ran towards them and deftly took their hands to stop them from falling, and they raced ahead of me, a perfect daisy chain, simple but complete, to the safety of the house. *This was how it will be, I thought. I will die and they will be together.* And they will be sad, but they will also laugh and be happy. And I will be dead, alone. I couldn't move. I started screaming silently.

Another time, I was sitting on the back step, watching the children as they splashed in the paddling pool. It was a bright day. I had to shield my eyes from the sun to see them clearly. I was sewing a fancy-dress costume for Cosima and I became aware of tears falling on to the cloth. Who would do this if I weren't here, I thought? And then I became angry. It's so fucking unfair that I have to think like this, I thought. And I rushed into the house to splash my face with cold water, to breathe deeply so that no one would know, so that I wouldn't upset anyone more than I already had.

Not all my misery was self-induced though. It was often caused by others, although usually not deliberately. After my diagnosis, people seemed to fall into distinct categories. Those who were closest to me – Simon, certain family members, Kerry and my friend Anna – were distressed by the news but transformed that distress into support. They were close enough to pitch into my life unselfconsciously. People who knew me less well were also distressed but confused as to what to say or do. Some managed to find a way through this confusion and were angels. They made me feel normal, part of the world when I felt I was falling off the edge. Others floundered around, often making me feel worse rather than better. 'Rather you than me' was one comment from a colleague. I was staggered by his insensitivity. The two smallest categories were the worst though. One consisted of those people who seemed to appear from nowhere, the ambulance chasers, the people whose names I hardly knew, but who suddenly seemed to know me well, who were exhilarated by my situation. The other consisted of those who seemed jealous of my situation, envious of the attention and sympathy it brought me. One work colleague told me that she was sick of people telling her what a tragedy my illness was. 'They've no idea how difficult it is working with someone who's had cancer,' she said. Another woman interrupted a story she was telling me about being rushed into hospital one weekend with, 'What's the point in telling you this? You can top any story.' A sub-section of this group were not so forceful in their outbursts. Their stories, everyday moans, simply trailed off as they suddenly worried that I couldn't possibly empathise with the fact that their life was in ruins because their car had broken down, the cat had gone missing. It was incredibly isolating.

I soon realised that while we are happy to talk about each other's broken legs or slipped discs, when we hear the word cancer, we are stunned, our manners desert us. It's obvious why. Cancer equals death to most of us – sometimes rightly, but often wrongly – and our generation, with its pill-for-everything mentality and peacetime presumptions, has a hard time dealing with mortality. A tactic I came across frequently was 'distancing'. Those who couldn't bear to contemplate the idea that it was simply bad luck that I had cancer tried to find a very specific reason why I had it and, therefore, why they wouldn't get it. It was often implied that it was my fault. A favourite comment was, 'You've always had such stressful jobs, it's not surprising.' Funny that the people I met at the clinic came from every background imaginable, including some who could only be described as bovine. But the most trying line was: 'Maybe you've been suppressing your anger.' I was sorely tempted to prove them wrong with a swift headbutt.

Lots and lots of people were inspired to tell me stories about friends, relations who had had cancer, the trouble they had had getting diagnosed, the horror of the treatment, how they never went back to work again, and so on. I never knew how to react to these stories. My sympathy reserves were low and the diagnoses and situations in these stories often bore no relevance to mine. More alarmingly, the stories often petered out as it suddenly dawned on the tellers that the punchline was that the person was now dead. Others couldn't bear to talk about cancer at all and would stop all discussion with: 'I just know you're going to be fine.' As my oncologist never said that to me, it was pretty galling to hear it from people who often would have been at a loss to explain exactly what an oncologist was. They often held up their hand as they spoke, like a traffic policeman, a bizarre way of telling me to stop, shut up, I don't want to hear this stuff.

The most extreme version of this tactic was complete denial – one acquaintance never mentioned my cancer, even when I was totally bald from chemotherapy. Others hid behind the post: you've no idea how insulting it is to get a card from a so-called friend asking you to get in touch when you're better. A much younger, former colleague wrote me a letter saying what an inspiration I had been to her and her generation. I'm sure it was well-intentioned but it read like an obituary. Whenever I went into my office, many of the men couldn't bring them-selves to mention what had happened to me. It felt awkward, almost surreal, but I couldn't be bothered to bring up the subject myself. It felt like one responsibility too many, so I let it ride.

By now you're probably thinking: 'But *I'm* not like that. *I* call a spade a spade.' This was preferable, of course, but not always entirely successful if not thought through. The editor of a women's magazine asked me if I would write an article for her about how cancer had destroyed my life and career. You know, she said, one minute I was a top journalist and now my life is over. A freelance writer I had lunch with breezily asked me, as the menu arrived, if I ever thought about death. 'All the time,' I wanted to say, 'but I don't want to talk about it in a noisy restaurant with a waiter hovering.' Nor did I want to talk about my prognosis in front of my children at the school gates, or on the phone when they were sitting two feet away happily playing.

More fun were the great advice givers. Apart from the diet-mongers, I was subject to frequent dissertations on the wonders of echinacea, carrot juice, coffee enemas and other natural remedies. My reaction was the same to them all. If the cure for cancer was available for a tenner at the local health food shop, I think the cancer czar would have been on to it by now. It would save the NHS a fortune.

Some people were saints though, always doing and saying the right thing. Most importantly, they said something quickly. They asked questions, too, as they would have done with any other problem. In short, they engaged with what was going on and treated me like a normal person, not a freak. Much later, I met people who felt guilty that they hadn't been in touch and it seemed that the longer they left it without contacting me, the more awkward they felt about it.

I also appreciated the people who didn't give up on me during those eight months of my treatment. It was a long haul and I was no fun. I often left the answerphone on when I was too depressed, tired or unwell to talk – and if I had answered all the calls, I would have been on the phone all the time – but it was comforting to know that people were rooting for me, particularly when they didn't expect a call back. Letters and cards ditto, as long as people weren't hiding behind them. Nowadays, it would be much easier with email and texting. I also loved getting presents. It really cheered me up. Not cancer books, but lipsticks, magazines, bath oil. Rebecca, Dee and Sue in the office were good at this. Life is doom-laden enough when you have cancer and I needed lightening up. Big time. Trivia made me feel normal.

I was grateful for offers of help, too. But – and it's a huge but – general, vague offers were hopeless, giving me something else to worry about, to organise. The most helpful people outside the inner circle were the self-starters. Janine always brought lunch when she visited, Penny ferried the children to and from a party, Paula tracked down information about my doctors for me, and Rosemary acted as the contact for anyone wanting an update so that I didn't have to keep repeating myself. She even told someone who kept ringing me, despite the fact that I hardly knew her, to leave me alone. These helpful people had taken to heart what Joe Slovo, the great anti-apartheid campaigner, said: 'I have cancer, but I also have feelings.'

The most potent help came from those who had been there before, who had had breast cancer themselves and, despite wanting to put the experience behind them as much as they could, took time to support me, cheer me on from the sidelines. They meant the world to me. Jackie, a friend of Simon's, talked to me about Mr Sinnett who had treated her and suggested questions for me to ask. Francine, as I have described, told me about the stem cell treatment. And then there was Katy. I had worked with Katy in my twenties, but had not seen her for about 15 years. Then I got a letter from her. It was in the hallway when we got back from the cottage one Sunday evening. She had had breast cancer herself, she said, and she wanted me to know that there was life after cancer. She also told me not to bother getting a wig if I lost my hair in chemo and that I could ring her any time. It was a short letter but my mood lifted from the basement to the top floor as I read it. All at once, I realised both how desperately lonely I had been feeling and how I wasn't so alone after all.

During treatment, I also met Shirley. I spotted her in Professor Coombes' clinic one day, a baby at her feet, and I forced myself on her. She was the only person I had ever seen there who looked even vaguely in the same age group as me. She was, in fact, younger and had been diagnosed when pregnant. We were, it turned out, both on the stem cell transplant trial and, when we met, both having our outpatient chemo. We started to meet up outside of the hospital and a kinship developed. I'm not sure how good we were for each other – we were both so traumatised and it was hard, at least for me, to look at her sometimes, to see in her face what I presume others saw in mine, a kind of madness. But it was wonderful to have someone with whom I could share the horror without feeling self-conscious or having to explain myself. Once the treatment was over though, our relationship was hard to maintain, its focus gone. This theme was played out elsewhere, too.

I was surrounded by sighs of relief. I had got through the worst, the treatment, was the general feeling. Soon I would be discharged from the hospital. The nightmare would be over. I had not died and normal service would be resumed. I had fought for my life and won. One phrase I heard often during this period was 'thank God that's over'. Another was 'well done'. I was told often how lucky I must feel, how I must leap out of bed each morning, glad to be alive. All these comments seemed to me, even in my fog, off the mark. I had a vague feeling that I hadn't actually done anything and that things were far from over. I felt as though my life had been saved, by Mr Sinnett and Professor Coombes and Dr Lowdell. My role had been some-what passive. I had endured the treatment rather than been in a fight or battle, that it had required a certain old-fashioned kind of fortitude of me rather than a gung-ho, nuke-the-bastards approach. And although I did feel lucky that I had not died, this fact somehow depressed me rather than filled me with joy. I felt demoted. I was now a person of whom little was expected.

Existence was, it seemed, my greatest achievement, something to crow about on my CV. I also seemed to be alone in wondering what would happen to me now. Whenever I brought up the subject, I felt as though I were making an unseemly fuss. It soon became obvious that I was moving in a different direction from everyone else. The message I was getting was that unhappiness was inappropriate now. The support melted, the presents and cards stopped. The party, such as it was, was over.

It is, I discovered later, a well-documented syndrome that the end of treatment is a difficult period for cancer patients. If we don't die, if our cancer seems, for the time being, to be under control, we experience a period of re-entry into the world, a reversal of the process by which we withdrew from it, and it is equally painful, perhaps more painful because it is not accompanied by numbness. The pain intensifies, in fact, as the numbness fades. We are confronted by a future when we thought we might not have one. But what does this future hold? It is not the same future we took for granted before our diagnoses. I didn't even know how to describe myself.

Another mother once told me a story. She had overheard her children talking about her.

'Mummy's got cancer,' said one.

'No, she used to have cancer,' said the other.

We laughed. That old chestnut, we said. She was, at that point, well. I had just finished treatment. Did we still have cancer or not? Most of us are not cured by our treatment. It carries no guarantees and the future is a question mark. And yet . . . There was a problem with the language. It hadn't caught up with modern life.

I'd come across this problem before I was ill. Simon and I had been together since I was 20, but we were not married and I never knew what to call him. I usually opted for 'partner' which sounded too business-like. It was also often misunderstood, as was the ambiguous 'father-of-my-children' which begged the question whether he was anything but a sperm donor, so sometimes I resorted to calling him my husband because it was easier. My friend Jane called him my boyfriend but that only worked when it was said in her ironic, knowing way. Lover was just way too smug and the other alternatives were just repulsive – significant other, other half, him indoors. The Australians opt for the term 'de facto spouse', shortening it to 'de facto', and when my Australian friend Linda was rushed into hospital during a trip to London with her partner Peter, nobody knew what it meant. Simon and I were sitting in the waiting room in casualty. A nurse appeared with a clipboard and asked for Mr De Facto. Nobody stirred. She asked again, and then suddenly Peter clicked. It was absurd, as absurd as my difficulties with describing the status of my cancer. It is a difficulty that has not gone away.

Some people used the term remission to describe my situation. It didn't feel right to me. It suggested that my cancer would definitely come back. It also suggested that my cancer had, for the moment, disappeared. The truth is that nobody knew if my cancer would come back or if I was harbouring a large number of cancer cells. The way I saw it was that my cancer had been put to sleep. It had spread to my lymph nodes, so it was highly likely that, alongside the obvious tumour in my breast, there were tiny, undetectable cancer cells swimming around in my system. Scans can only detect tumours. In my unscientific analysis, the surgery and radiotherapy dealt with the tumour and the brutal chemotherapy rendered the breakaway cells unconscious which meant, of course, that they could recover at some point, go forth and multiply. In the best of all possible worlds, the chemo killed them, but nobody knew for sure.

Meanwhile I was abandoned to a linguistic limbo-land. Did I or did I not have cancer? The most accurate way of describing my situation is that I am living with cancer. It's good, the best there is, the 'partner' of cancer terminology, but it doesn't work when you come up to me and ask me how I am. I'm not sure I could actually say the words, 'Oh, you know, living with cancer.' In this book, I describe my cancer experience in phases. I use the phrase 'when I was diagnosed' to describe, well, when I was diagnosed with cancer. I use the phrase 'when I was ill' to describe the eight-month period when I was having treatment for that cancer. I use the phrase 'after treatment' to describe the period immediately following my radiotherapy. I have not, however, come up with a phrase I feel comfortable with for the last six years. When I was discussing this book with my friend Tim and throwing around ideas for titles, I mentioned that I had been reading Virginia Woolf's *On Being Ill* and how I was considering the title *On Not Being Ill*. Tim suggested *On Not Being Dead*. I like both. Neither works in conversation though.

Some people like the word survivor, as in I am a cancer survivor. It's a legacy of the self-help movement, as in I am an incest survivor. It's not bad. I use it occasionally. But I couldn't until fairly recently. I wasn't sure that I could. When do you officially become a survivor? At two years, three years? Is there some etiquette involved? I still don't know.

There are many phrases and words that just trip off the tongue in conversations about cancer though. The most common way to describe cancer treatment and cancer research is by using military terminology. Scientists are waging a war on cancer. Patients battle cancer and, in obituaries, have lost their battle with cancer. Cancer is the enemy. It is a stealth bomb, we don't hear it coming. Discussing my stem cell transplant, the phrase ground zero was used. The day after my immune system was considered destroyed by the high-dose chemo was called Day One. Chemotherapy itself is often described as carpet-bombing. People who get involved in visual imagery, imagining their cancer cells being overcome in some way – the idea being that if you can imagine something, it can really happen – usually end up becoming military strategists, conjuring up images of generals and tanks and scud missiles. I had always thought visual imagery was nonsense but I had a go. At first, all I could come up with was an image of a vacuum cleaner sweeping up the cancer cells, which was rather tame and uninteresting as I wield a vacuum cleaner about three times a year. I came up with a better image when I was in Shropshire where I like to go out into the garden last thing at night and look at the stars – I can't see many in London. I rather liked the idea of cancer cells flowing out of my body and up into the Milky Way. I couldn't go with the military flow.

I still can't and, as I started to try to make sense of my experience, I discovered that my view of cancer was different in other ways from most people's. Cancer, to me, is a disease and nothing else. I have moments of paranoia when I feel otherwise, but generally, for me, cancer has no wider meaning. It is not evil. It is not cunning. It does not have a mind of its own in any way. It is simply a disease which is imperfectly understood by the medical profession. Many people find this unacceptable though and, faced with this void of knowledge, fill it with fantasies about cancer's power, imagine it as all-powerful. They feel defensive, the need to get out the big guns. They don't talk about heart disease like this, or any other disease. AIDS came in for the apocalyptic treatment briefly, but it's cancer that frightens most, remains synonymous with death, preceded by terrible destruction. Once the knowledge gap is closed, all this will fall away. Cancer will become, as it should be now, just another disease. But for now, it is invested with such strength that it seems imperative to talk big back. It's big willy talk, ridiculous, and makes anyone with cancer feel much worse than they need to.

This is why. When you are diagnosed with cancer, you are inundated with advice about fighting it – not, it has to be said, by doctors. However, the form this fight should take is left rather vague. What is made clear though is that if you don't fight, you will die and it will be your fault, just as it is probably your fault that you got the cancer in the first place. It's clutching at straws – nobody knows why many people get cancer. But ambiguity and uncertainty are so uncomfortable that it's easier to blame the person with cancer – or victim or sufferer as they are often, melodramatically, called. She was too inhibited, angry, stressed, generally too uptight and, well, all this stuff has to come out somewhere and, such a shame, but it's hardly surprising, it's come out as cancer and if she doesn't get a better attitude, she's going to die. It's another version of she-shouldn't-have-gone-out-in-that-short-skirt.

One day, we shall look back and laugh at the assumptions that are made about cancer today, its causes and treatment, in the same way that we laugh about doctors using leeches and the romantic spin around tuberculosis. It may take some time though. Susan Sontag wrote her essay about cancer called *Illness as Metaphor* exploring some of these ideas back in 1977. Most of her conclusions are still pertinent today.

Meanwhile we should mind our language. We should junk the military jargon. We should admit how little we know about cancer, how much that scares us and how it might make us use certain words and phrases unkindly. We should also stop using the word cancer as a metaphor for every nasty, creeping thing in the world. As Susan Sontag points out, the word cancer, although it comes from the Greek and Latin words for crab, was probably chosen for the disease not because it creeps or crawls like a crab through the body, but because the swollen veins of an external tumour look like a crab's legs, a sight modern surgery and drugs thankfully save most of us from nowadays.

As I started to grapple with these issues back in 1998, I often felt overwhelmed, defeated, so, instead, I tried to focus on getting back to normal. I genuinely believed that if I tried hard enough I would be able to and, if I could, it would give me some kind of peace. After all, the people around me seemed to be doing just that. I threw myself back into office life. I tried to recreate my pre-illness routines. Superficially, I was quite successful, but underneath, I was confused, my every step dogged by nagging doubts about my life which, however much it looked the same, did not feel the same. And I found myself drained of energy by the depressing thought that, with such a huge question mark over my future, was there really any point in making all this effort. I felt totally unable to plan ahead. Often I couldn't think about tomorrow, let alone next week, next month, a summer holiday, Christmas.

The point of my life might seem obvious. I had two children. I had a partner. I had family, friends, a good job. But the trauma of my diagnosis and treatment was so powerful that, once I started to try and examine and make sense of what had happened to me, I also found myself examining my whole life. Dr Lowdell's question about how I was coping haunted me. The experience of having cancer, I began to realise, had shaken my confidence in a profound way. I felt disconnected. I felt too weird, too heavy, serious, humourless. I felt both unable to recreate my old life and unable to go forward. One evening, I went to a work dinner at the Groucho Club. I hated every single minute of it. Everyone was nice to me, but I couldn't relax. I hated everyone round the table simply because they did not have cancer. I could not bear to hear them laughing and joking. I was diminished by my envy of their seemingly carefree lives. I went home feeling terrified that this loneliness, this anger and misery would be my lot now.

I needed to learn how to do something, I thought. I wasn't sure what it was, but I knew it was something I would have to do alone. I started reading. I have a talent for reading. Maybe it's my greatest talent. Both the flat and our cottage are full of books, crammed into bookshelves, piled up on the stairs. They slide around on bedside tables, spilling on to the floor. When I go on holiday, I pack one book for each day. Given the choice, I'd rather read a book than do most other things. The hardest aspect of having small children for me was not being able to read. I was too exhausted at night and, in the day, I had to watch them every minute. I didn't miss going out. I didn't mind being covered in goo. I didn't really care that I had to go to bed at 10pm because I had to get in some sleep before the awakenings began. I hated not being able to read though and one of the benefits of being ill was that I had time to do so again.

I couldn't read when I was very ill, but I could at home when the nausea or pain was more background than foreground. In fact, it was the only thing I could do as I couldn't bear watching TV during the day even in my most miserable moments. I started reading in a way that I hadn't since my twenties, for hours and hours at a time. I also joined the library in a moment of panic about money. I signed up at my local branch, a tiny library in the Brompton Road which the children belonged to. I roamed the shelves, reading randomly, released from the pressure of keeping up, the bane of every journalist's life.

On a deeper level, it reminded me of different times in my life. When I was a child, we went to the library every week. I belonged to a Good Readers club. Now I suddenly remembered working my way through volumes of folk tales from different countries. I also remembered what it felt like when I first joined the adult library, how confused I was, lugging home baffling books in which people called each other hon and had relationships. 'What's a hon?' I asked my mother, pronouncing it like hot.

I remembered how proud I was to get a Saturday job at the library when I was 15, a serious step up from the jobs I'd had in Kiddie City, a local toy shop where I'd prowled the aisles supposedly looking for shoplifters, and Boots, where I'd worn a nylon overall and filled shelves. At Boots I'd got a discount and stocked up on cheap make-up, but now I had a better perk – I could take out as many books as I liked. And I did, taking home piles each Saturday evening on the bus. I joined the picture library, something which seems to have disappeared now, and took home paintings for the week. They must have been terrible reproductions, but I thought they were fabulous, great art.

Then there were the memories of revising for my A-levels in the library, dreaming quietly in a booth, staring at the moody black and white photograph of Camus with his fag on my Penguin paperback of *La Peste* and wondering if I would ever inhabit such a glamorous world. At university it was different. The library was a palace compared to the local library and a place I visited often at first. But it was all about sex then, checking out the boys – you couldn't really call them men – and the coffee bar. What all these experiences had in common though was a sense of possibility and this rose up in me again when I joined the Brompton Library. Tentatively, though, for what were the possibilities now?

But I was unable to find any books in the library to help me. Books to pass the time, yes. Books to enjoy, yes. But books to guide me, no. I started buying self-help books, something I had never done before. I couldn't find any about what it felt like to survive a cancer diagnosis, so I ploughed my way through a few general feel-the-fear type books. Oh Lord. Most I threw away, something I had also never done before. They were mainly drivel and unmemorable, leaving me with the feeling that I had somehow made myself ill and could therefore will myself better, which made no sense at all. The ones I do remember and so presume were less ghastly, less glib, were *The Road Less Travelled* by M. Scott Peck, Harriet Lerner's *The Dance of Anger* and *Women's Bodies, Women's Wisdom* by Christine Northrup. Even so, they were books I would not have touched with a bargepole had I not been so desperate and they were of no help whatsoever. Eventually, I avoided any book that mentioned the words chakra or self-healing.

I was briefly waylaid by *The Tibetan Book of Living and Dying*, finding solace in its acceptance of death, but I abandoned it at the first mention of reincarnation. Edmund White's *Farewell Symphony*, a novel about New York during the height of the AIDS crisis, was comforting. The elegiac quality of the book moved me, tapped into my own confused feelings about the unfairness of life, the horror of facing mortality too soon, the strangeness of survival. Later, I found *PWA*, the book of Oscar Moore's AIDS diary, helpful, too. There was something about the experience of AIDS at that time which resonated with me, the outrage, the loneliness, the unspeakable treatment. I could not, however, read Ruth Picardie's column about dying from breast cancer which was running in the *Observer* when I was diagnosed and which was later turned into a book. It felt too close to home, too grim. I wasn't ready for that; resisted the idea that I would ever be ready for it. Later, I occasionally read John Diamond's column in the *Times* about his experience of throat cancer and I did read his book *C: Because cowards get cancer too*. I had worked with John, knew him and we occasionally emailed each other. He was a clever writer, funny, and he broke down many taboos, but I couldn't relate to his larky tone. I was way too gloomy.

I had yet to discover Virginia Woolf's *On Being Ill*, Susan Sontag's *Illness as Metaphor* or Joan Didion's eponymous essay in *The White Album*, all of which are works of the highest order about the experience of disconnection and which I have now read many times. Back then, I was flailing around. I struck lucky when I tried reading serious, rather than self-help, books with a psychological bent. Some were dry, but Adam Phillips' were mesmerising. I drank in his words, feeling excited, exhilarated. Here was someone who understood, I felt. But as I finished each book, I went blank. What had he said? I couldn't say and I can't now. I think though that his books spoke to me, gave me a sense, albeit inchoate, that there was another language to describe what I was feeling and that acquiring it was some kind of key. All I had to do now was find out what this language was. It took some time.

5

Ray Of Light

I stumbled into therapy, or at least that's what I thought at the time. Now, six years on, I know much more about psychology. I now know that there are probably no such things as accidents, although initially that's what it felt like. It was true at the time and that's fine because one of the other things I have learned over the years is that what I think is subject to change. Each day brings new perspectives which don't necessarily make what I thought yesterday or last year untrue, merely what I thought at that time, what I *could* think at the time. It is, however, an unacceptable way of thinking to most people. There is an obsession with pinning things down, getting at The Truth. As was I back in 1998. I was determined to nail this cancer thing.

I had never thought about going into therapy. I'd never dismissed it. I had friends who had found it helpful. But I never thought about it for myself, in the same way that I had never thought about playing rugby. It was nowhere on my wish list. It presented itself to me as an option, almost by fluke it seemed, and I decided to pursue it.

Now, as I said, I know a fair amount about psychology. I have read books about it. I took a Birkbeck course on the subject. I am familiar with the terminology – transference, countertransference, Oedipus complex, resistance, the false self, seduction theory, etc., etc. I have strong views on what I think about various types of therapy – if you care about such things, I think, rather conventionally, that Freud was a genius and I greatly admire Carl Rogers. But this information I now have is, in so many ways, irrelevant. Interesting, but irrelevant. The only point about therapy, for me, is the experience of therapy. The insights come from the therapy, not reading a book about it. It's not such a radical idea. You can read a book about how to ride a bicycle and then, faced with a real bicycle, fall straight off. And so you can read a hundred books about therapy, psychology, analysis, and fail to have one single meaningful insight about your own behaviour. Back in 1998, though, I knew nada, either in theory or in practice.

When I was briefly depressed as a student, my GP sent someone – I have no idea who – to see me at home. He arrived unannounced at the flat I shared with two other girls one Saturday morning, walked into the bathroom where one of them was having a bath and, when he eventually found his bearings and me, studied my bookshelves and suggested that I felt depressed because I was reading too many gloomy books. One such misery-inducer seemed to be *One Hundred Years of Solitude*. Tell that to my tutors, I thought. He said I could arrange to go and talk to him if I wanted. I didn't. I recovered, naturally it seemed, under my own steam after a couple of days' recuperation at my parents'. I never felt that depressed again or curious enough about myself to consider therapy. I had seen the counsellor at Charing Cross while I was waiting for my stem cell transplant, but I had seen her for a purpose, I felt, which was to deal with my specific fears about my treatment, and not for depression as such. I saw her just three or four times. I therefore date my therapy from my first session with Sally Parr at the Cromwell in January 1998. It took me a while to realise that's what it was, though.

That January, as I was starting my radiotherapy treatment, I picked up a leaflet from the reception desk while I was waiting to check in for my appointment. Normally there was no one else at the desk, but that day there was a queue, so I passed the time looking at the information leaflets. The hospital, it seemed, offered 12 cancer counselling sessions during treatment. I put the flyer in my bag. A couple of days later, I decided to make an appointment. I'm not sure why. I didn't really know what the term 'cancer counselling' meant, I just had an instinct that it might help me understand why I was so depressed. But I didn't have particularly high hopes for it. I hadn't been looking for a therapist. The deciding factor was that the sessions were free, thrown in with my radiotherapy. Such is the casual way that important decisions are made. Perhaps. Because, of course, I had been bombarded with advice from friends about diet, crystals, positive thinking, given telephone numbers for this, that and the other expert or course. I'd received printouts from cancer organisations about support groups. There were so many courses of action I could have pursued at that time, but I didn't. I chose to pursue the cancer counselling.

There were two therapists at the hospital and mine was to be Sally Parr. I am so glad it was. I could have ended up with anyone, some glorified aromatherapist, someone who'd done a correspondence course in counselling, someone who could have done more harm than good. But I got Sally Parr.

The first session was easy, at first. Sally asked me to tell her about myself, which I took to mean telling her about my diagnosis and treatment. Once I'd started, I couldn't stop: and then, and then, and then . . . I was on a roll. I can do this, I thought. And then she said that my dilemma was finding a way to hope, but not too much. And then I couldn't speak. She had said what I couldn't admit to myself and what nobody else seemed able to say to me in so many words. It was the nub of the matter, what I had been wrestling with. I had expected her to comment on my treatment, respond to something specific I had said, perhaps give me advice. Instead, she drew my attention to the bigger picture. It was so bloody obvious. But that, I was to learn, was what therapy would be like for me. I would waffle on about something, then the therapist would say a few words, not many usually, and usually not in response to any of the detail of my monologues. I would be completely taken aback by the pertinence of the comments. Of course, I would say. That's it, exactly. I would, however, also feel infuriated that I had been unable to see whatever it was for myself. I frequently felt completely stupid.

This comment about hope had a similar effect on me to Simon's comment, when I was first diagnosed, about there being no going back. It forced me to look at where I was, rather than where I had been. And where was that exactly? It also shone a torch on my new relationship with mortality. On one level, I did know what I was grappling with, but only dimly, and I had little confidence even in that dim comprehension. It was difficult to think about what I really felt, with everyone else so confident that I was now on the road to recovery, that it, my cancer, was over, that we could all go back to normal now. Perhaps they didn't believe it either, but they said it anyway, perhaps needed to say it. I couldn't agree, but I didn't seem to be able to articulate a convincing case for the opposition. The problem seemed too vague, too so-what. Every time I tried to think about the ambiguity of my situation, that fog would descend and I would hear a voice, a perfectly rational voice, saying, we've all got to die sometime. What's new? Any one of us – and this is a phrase I have grown to loathe – could get run over by a bus tomorrow. But, apart from the fact that, at this time, I had never, ever heard of anyone being run over by a bus, I knew that before I was diagnosed with cancer, I had never felt as unsure and confused about the future as I did now.

In that first session with Sally, I saw clearly how I could talk about my diagnosis and treatment, in a superficial way, with ease. I could not talk about today or tomorrow, superficially or any other way, because I could not imagine my own future. I was stuck, that rabbit in the headlights. I couldn't move, haunted, immobilised by that question – how could I carry on, knowing that each day I might wake up and my cancer would be back.

I wasn't being melodramatic. I knew the facts, that my cancer could come back at any time, the usual places being the liver, lungs or bones, and that treatment for advanced cancer came with even fewer guarantees. I knew that scans cannot detect tiny cancer cells, that I was likely to experience symptoms before they detected anything. When I had finished my treatment, I had had a sobering conversation with Professor Coombes.

'So what do I do now then?' I said.

'Sorry?' he said, worrying his stethoscope, the high priest in his all-knowing white coat, but with only the truth of *uncertainty* to offer a supplicant like me. No easy way out for him, no pat little tales of everlasting life.

'What do I do now?' I said again.

He looked at me, sort of. 'Well,' he said. 'We'll make an appointment for you to come back in three months.'

'No. I mean, what do I *do*?'

He glanced out of the window. 'Do? You don't need to *do* anything.'

'But what's going to happen to me?'

He looked at me, carefully this time. 'I don't know.'

'Am I going to be all right?' It was my turn to look away.

'I don't know. You've had all the treatment, and now we just have to wait and see what happens.'

I knew this already, of course. But I wanted a different answer. There were two other possible answers and I wanted to hear one of them now. I knew I wouldn't though – couldn't, the facts got in the way – and that I would spend the rest of my life preparing and waiting to hear the other.

'Do you think I should take vitamins?' I said.

'See you in three months,' he said.

I had, of course, never been told I would be okay. I wasn't told I would not be okay, but the ambivalence had been there from the beginning with my doctors, in the form of silences, non-answers to questions, phrases such as 'we will do our best' and 'we will do what we can'. The anaesthetist who had assisted on my mastectomy was more direct. When I rang him to sort out a bill for my insurance, he asked me how I was and said he was sorry, that they always hoped for the best and sometimes when they operated it turned out to be worse than they had thought. Such bad luck, he said. He wished me well, but he sounded unconvinced that wellness was on the cards for me. Professor Coombes had been direct, in a different way, when he talked to me about my chemotherapy and described me as being, for the moment, in a category in which I could be helped. The message was clear: the future looks doubtful. But I found it hard to absorb this information, this ambiguity. It was like trying to bottle mercury.

This ambiguity is not the fault of the doctors. They rarely know what the future holds. In some situations, when cancer has spread widely, is inoperable or not responding to treatment, then they probably can say with some degree of confidence that your number's up. But even then they aren't always right. People can die faster than predicted or much more slowly. And, as Professor Coombes once explained to me, patients who are expected to do well sometimes don't, and vice versa. It's hardly surprising that they mainly reserve judgement.

I played games with my own judgement, too. Around this time, I did ask, repeatedly, if I was going to be okay. I repeatedly got the answer I expected: 'We don't know.' But I didn't ask about statistics. I looked at a book in Waterstone's once which contained a graph showing breast cancer survival rates. It was a downward slope with steep declines at certain points. I can't remember when these points occurred – after three years, five years – because I snapped the book shut. I didn't want to know.

I also never asked for my exact diagnosis. I was told that I had lobular breast cancer, as opposed to the more common ductal carcinoma, but I never asked for its stage. Staging is the way in which tumours are graded, stage one being mild, stage four being terminal. There are grades within those stages. Some people like to bandy about this kind of information about their cancer. They are almost boastful. But I feel I'm better off not knowing. The general gist is bad enough and that little area of haziness makes me feel that there are still possibilities for me. Knowing would feel like the drawbridge being drawn up, imprisoning me in the castle while life went on over the other side of the moat. Maybe if I did ask, you're probably thinking, I'd be pleasantly surprised. Maybe. But maybe not. It's a risk I don't want to take. To me, it's the difference between dicing with life and dicing with death.

As I left the Cromwell after that first session with Sally, I felt that I had taken a small step towards finding the language to articulate my confusion, to explain why I was so depressed. But I was crying. I was exhausted. I felt worse, not better. Something wrong here, I thought. She may have been right, but did I want to hear this stuff? I decided to go back the following week, but was wary. This time, Sally waited for me to start talking. I did not find it difficult. I have heard of people who do, who spend their therapeutic hour in silence, but I have never had this problem, not once. I did, however, still expect Sally to start, after a while, making suggestions, giving me advice. She didn't. When I paused, she didn't leap in, she waited. When I cried, she didn't try to comfort or stop me. The weirdness was starting. Somewhere along the line, though, she asked me if I felt angry. Of course not, I said. What was the point of being angry? Who was I supposed to be angry with? What had happened to me wasn't fair, but then life isn't fair. And, anyway, talking about cancer being unfair is silly, it's the language of the playground. It wasn't as if it was anyone's fault that I had cancer. Sally didn't argue with me, just listened. A few days later, I was walking along the street and suddenly felt overwhelmed by the realisation that I *was* angry, extremely angry. Tears rolled down my face and I didn't care. This is so unfair, I muttered bitterly. And, much to my amazement, my head felt clearer.

Was I just incredibly suggestible? Was this a case of the situation being obvious to everyone but me? The answer is probably yes to both questions. But the point is that nobody had ever asked me before if I was angry and I couldn't see that I was. The question allowed me to see that I was, and once I could see it, I could stop resisting it and that, in turn, made me feel better, lighter. Simple really. Money for old rope perhaps. Except that I had been asked many, many questions before: the wrong questions. This was the right question, the therapeutic question. It was an extraordinary experience for me, to come to an understanding, to learn something in a way that had nothing to do with books and swotting and the intellect and nailing things down. It seemed to be all about doing nothing, allowing my mind to go into freefall, holding back on the rational arguments, the intellectual justifications, so that the true emotions and feelings, grey and contradictory, could float into my consciousness.

But this is something I understood only vaguely at the time. From a distance of six years, I can look back and see my therapy as a series of such breakthroughs leading to a version of enlightenment, rather like that TV ad for jeans in which two people crash through wall after wall to freedom. It sounds exhilarating, but exhilaration came later. For a long time, the breakthroughs felt, at best, like relief and, the rest of the time, I felt like shit. I would sit in the sessions, rambling and crying. I would go home, red-faced and exhausted, and fall instantly asleep. I tried to write down what I had talked about and possibly learned and, when I read back my notes later, they were nonsense. And yet, even in this fog, after only a couple of sessions with Sally I knew that I had found what I was looking for. I also realised that what she was practising, with me, was not so much counselling as therapy and therapy with an analytic bent. It suited me well.

After the 12 free sessions, I wanted more and started paying to see Sally once and sometimes twice a week. I had realised that although I had learned something about my feelings about having cancer, I had a long way to go. One day in May, however, Sally announced that she was going on maternity leave. I was shocked. How could she possibly be pregnant? It was obvious when I looked at her carefully, but I had been so self-absorbed that I hadn't noticed. What else hadn't I noticed, I wondered?

She said that if I wanted to continue, I could see the person who would be replacing her or she could refer me to someone outside the hospital. This was a difficult decision because I realised that going to the hospital each week for my therapy had been a bonus. I was still, in some way, connected to the hospital, under its auspices. It was a comfort blanket. I knew I had to learn to live without it. But I was also worried about finding a proper, trained therapist. Sally suggested she refer me to Anna Witham who she thought I might be able to work with. I went for an introductory session in the June to see if I liked her and if she could or would take me on (I'm still not entirely sure who was assessing who). I was to go back to Sally afterwards to discuss the session.

I went along from work one sunny lunchtime, full of trepidation, to Anna Witham's flat – or what I presume is her flat because I have absolutely no idea whether or not she lives there. It was in a mansion block. I rang the bell on the main door, was let in, then, when nobody appeared when I reached the flat door, I rang the flat bell and was buzzed into a small, empty hallway. Bemused, I sat down on the little chair and looked around. I was confronted by four identical doors. A woman then swept through one of them and led me through another which turned out to be two doors, one bang against the other, I presumed for sound-proofing. The room was small and comfortable. She sat on a lounger-style chair. I was asked if I wanted to sit on the chair opposite her or lie on the couch. *A couch? Oh my goodness.* I chose the chair. There was a bookshelf in the corner – I glimpsed an edition of Freud – and there were discreet prints on the walls. There was an oriental rug on the floor and, as I discovered later, a table to the left of my chair on which perched a box of tissues. Mrs Witham as I came to call her – for no reason I can discern apart from the fact that it says Mrs Anna Witham on her headed paper – looked ten or so years older than me. So that was good. She wouldn't be going on maternity leave. She seemed to be more intelligent than me. So that was good, too. She was elegantly dressed and quietly spoken which was pleasing. But the clinchers were that she seemed unafraid and on the wall was a drawing by Kathe Kollwitz, an artist I admire. This could work, I thought. And it did.

She didn't, I realise, say much that first session, but one of the things she did say shocked me. I asked her what Sally had told her about me. I knew by then that therapists rarely answer direct questions, but Mrs Witham came straight back at me. Sally, she said, felt I needed somewhere to be depressed. I'm not sure what I expected to hear. Something specific about the trauma I had been through, I suppose, my psychological state, perhaps how interesting I was. But there it was: a simple need to be allowed to moan once a week for 50 minutes. It was true though and it is true of much therapy.

There was no one else who could bear to listen to me drone on and on, and even if they could, I did not feel that it was right or fair to inflict my meanderings on others. How many times could I subject Simon to evenings of gloom and misery as I recounted my sorrows? How could I endlessly describe things he had seen with his own eyes? He had, after all, been with me for so much of the time. He was also, like so many others, trying to recover now, trying to move on. I felt not only confused and embarrassed that I seemed to be going backwards instead of forwards, but guilty that I was not bucking up. I did not want to be a burden any more. But once I understood how therapy helped me, it felt entirely appropriate to use it cathartically. For one hour a week, I could let rip. The process was important, but so was the knowledge that, whatever came up, that hour was there for *me* and it allowed me, for much of the time, to have a more normal, less doom-laden home and work life. There is obviously more to therapy than this, but it is wrong to ignore the benefits of just being listened to in a non-judgemental way. Some people even go as far as to say that it is the main benefit. I'm not so sure about that, but it is human nature to interrupt, reassure, to have a dialogue. The quality of the listening in therapy is quite different. It is not only seemingly inexhaustible, but so powerful that it elicits a different response, both more formal and more rambling, from ordinary conversation. I have often been amazed by what I say in the sessions. *Where did that come from?* I have been taken aback by what I have ended up talking about when I had every intention of talking about something else. I have had to come to terms with the fact that I start where I have to.

When I first met Mrs Witham though, I realised that I had a lot to learn about the basic mechanics of therapy. At the Cromwell, sessions had sometimes run over to accommodate my distress. I had been able to change my appointment times easily. I soon realised that I had been protected from a host of rules. The first is that therapists tend not to work in August (hence the jokes, in certain circles, about summer madness), so I would have to wait until September to start my therapy with Mrs Witham. I was also given a regular, weekly slot. I might be able to change it, I was told, but not necessarily. If I missed a session, for whatever reason – illness, work – I would have to pay for it. I would even have to pay when I went on holiday, but there would be no sessions when Mrs Witham was away – August, a few weeks at Easter and Christmas. The sessions would last 50 minutes exactly. If I was late, the time would not be made up. If I was upset at the end of a session, I would still have to leave (although there have been occasions when Mrs Witham has bent that rule a little). These restrictions infuriated me. Was Mrs Witham a complete control freak, I wondered? Another problem that emerged was my own attitude to therapy. When I was seeing Sally, it was easy for me to see the therapy as a continuation of my treatment. I could almost convince myself that I had not chosen it, pass it off as part of the general protocol, see and portray myself as the patient, following instructions. Seeing Mrs Witham was different and I suddenly felt self-conscious about my choice. It felt odd paying for support, almost shameful, an admission of failure. Peter, the editor of the paper, very kindly allowed me to leave early on Mondays for my sessions – it would have been very difficult to find the time otherwise – but one of my other bosses used to find it very amusing that I was in therapy. 'Meet Kate,' she'd say. 'She's mad.'

Very quickly, however, the pros outweighed the cons. The rules that I disliked, I soon realised, were helpful. The time restriction concentrated my mind, gave the sessions a soothing rhythm, and I knew, in the clearest of ways, that they were not endless, which would have been daunting. The commercial aspect made me take the process more seriously and freed me from reciprocating support, the way I would in a normal conversation, by empathising, listening, entertaining. I could be totally selfish when I was with Mrs Witham. It was liberating. I could, for 50 minutes a week, think about myself. Some people think this is self-indulgent. If it is, it's a uniquely puritanical form of self-indulgence. I had fallen down a well and I was trying to get myself out. Mrs Witham was the rope thrown down, but it was me, week after week, bracing myself against the walls and trying to clamber to the top again. It was hard work.

At first, I had an insatiable desire to describe to Mrs Witham the trauma of my treatment. In some ways, I seemed to be suffering from post-traumatic stress. I told her repeatedly what had happened to me during those eight months, each time remembering different things, different horrors. Each telling was disturbing, exhausting. So why did I do it? The telling was compulsive. It felt like a natural process, necessary. It made my experience feel real and justified, in some ways, the trauma I felt. Once my treatment was over, it seemed to quickly fade in most people's memories. Sometimes this made me feel as if it had never happened, that I had imagined it. Many people, I realised, were completely unaware that I had had radiotherapy and one woman described my chemotherapy as one of life's little hurdles before changing the subject to the new boots she had just bought.

The repeated telling also enabled me to re-experience the trauma, with feeling, which sounds masochistic but was useful. Just because I went through my treatment in a state of numbness, it didn't mean that I had no feelings about it. I did, but these feelings were buried under layers of denial and shock. I was now able to feel those feelings. This was traumatic, too. But somehow the process completed a circle, married the two experiences, the physical and the emotional. It enabled me to see the experience for what it was for me – a profound disruption of the story I told myself about my life – not what it was supposed to be or what anyone else, doctors, my family, friends, so-called experts, thought it was. As I did this, I was able gradually to accept and absorb it, and tentatively move forward in a real, rather than a superficial way.

An unlooked-for side-effect of this painful process is that I find that I now feel things more keenly as they happen. For example, a few years ago, I agreed to take part in a trial at Charing Cross for a breast cancer screening test, a holy grail of sorts. It involved having my bone marrow taken every six months. As I write, it is ongoing. The first couple of times I went along, I had the procedure, which is ghastly and painful, then went straight into work. I would then feel out of sorts for the rest of the week without understanding why. Then I started going straight home to bed. I faced up to the way it upset me immediately and, apart from a sore bum, I felt fine the next day. I admitted that I found it painful as the needle went in, disturbing when I felt the clunk as it went into my bone, unsettled by the rummaging deep inside my body. I admitted that it made me angry. It was a small change and I'm not sure I could maintain this presence of mind during a real crisis, but it's an important one. It's apparent during the good times, too, because, much to my surprise, I also enjoy the good times more now. I think that when you suppress the lows, you also suppress the highs. All the emotions get flattened.

I have, so far, seen Mrs Witham for nearly six years. It's a long time. Perhaps. We live in an age of the quick-fix, where we want a remedy, a solution to our problems fast. One of the most popular forms of therapy nowadays is cognitive therapy which sometimes takes place over just six sessions. Maybe it works for some people. Maybe it's what's affordable. I did something different, I don't regret one minute of it and I'll stop going when I stop going, when it's no longer helpful. I have, of course, not spent all that time talking about my cancer. I have talked about other aspects of my life. What I have learned about myself is important, but only to me. The detail is of no relevance to anyone else at all. You are not me. However, there are themes which may be of interest to anyone in crisis. As Simon has often commented, what I have been through is what everyone is going through but they don't realise until a disaster happens. I certainly wish I had had a firmer grasp of these themes when I was ill.

One is that I reacted to having cancer as I reacted to everything in my life. I did not become a different person when I was diagnosed. I am pragmatic, I act when faced with difficult situations and I am incredibly organised. That coping mechanism worked when I was well – I held down a demanding job and ran two homes with relative ease – and it worked often enough when I was in treatment for me to think it was a runner. There was plenty to organise and do, after all. It failed me when I came out of treatment, though, when there was no longer anything obvious to do about my situation. What I then did, of course, was to go into therapy, an action of sorts, but an action which has taught me that action is not always possible and that I have to find another way forward.

Out of this came the knowledge that I, like everyone else, am doomed to repeat myself. If something worked for me in the past, I will try it again and again, despite all evidence to the contrary that it still works. I was, for example, a control freak in the sense that I thought that if I tried hard enough, I could control certain aspects of my life – in particular, how I spent my time and the kind of work I did, a useful quality in journalism, which thrives on the battle of wills, but useless when you have cancer. I also learned that I sometimes saw the world in black and white, in terms of either/or, again a useful tool in a newspaper office, completely useless as a way of understanding a complex experience like having cancer where there is rarely a right or wrong way to proceed, just many options, compromises and a surprise round every corner. This has been particularly hard for me to accept, that there are no answers, no certainties; just possibilities.

Therapy helped me see these and many other patterns of behaviour – none of them terribly rare or exciting, but nonetheless unhelpful – and understand where they came from. This knowledge then enabled me to stop repeating myself. I am not always successful. I am frequently a bit slow at realising what I'm up to. I can still feel angry about the fact that no one is ever going to sit me down and reassure me or tell me exactly what is going to happen to me. I would not say that I have replaced these patterns with others either, more that I try not to have knee-jerk reactions to situations. I have also learned to see what triggers anxiety in me, so that I feel specific anxiety rather than the more frightening, free-floating kind. It may not sound like much, but it is.

I could not have seen these patterns myself. I had glimpsed them in the past, but I had not fully understood them. It was painful realising how predictable my behaviour was and how it sometimes hindered me. It took painstaking work to unearth its roots. But it has been worth it. I'm not sure that anyone else can see the difference. I have not as such changed. But I feel different. I feel more myself and that self is a slightly different self from the self I was when I went into therapy and the self I was before I was ill. This, for me, is strange because I went into therapy feeling unhappy and missing my old self, and what has happened is that I have become a new self. And happier. I call that a result.

Therapy-bashing is a popular pastime now. The talk of us living in an age of counselling and the notion that Princess Diana was responsible for making the British more emotionally engaged is garbage. Mainly, you hear people laughing about counselling, therapy. If you're burgled, you hear the chortles. *Did they give you the victim support leaflet?* When there's a rail crash, you hear them, too. *Bet they'll all get counselling. What a waste of money.* They sneer at what is seen as the American love affair with self-improvement, at famous devotees of analysis such as Woody Allen – which is a nonsense because if you actually talk to Americans, they are just as hostile to the notion of therapy as we are. It's only in New York and California that it is more socially acceptable. People are ashamed of needing help, seeking help and being in therapy. From the beginning I have been open about having therapy, even when, at the beginning, I felt so self-conscious about it. But I have been astounded by the number of people who have since confessed to me that they were in therapy, too, but never told anyone, and I am always being asked how I found my therapist, what therapy is like. These questions are asked in hushed tones when there is no one else around. The conversations have the air of a dodgy drug deal.

I am careful what I say. Therapy is not the answer to all our problems. Some therapists are dreadful, dangerous. Therapy is also expensive. But – and this is a huge but – I do believe that therapy has helped me. I also believe that if we were taught as children about the way in which our minds work, about our emotions, our motivations and neuroses, in the same way that we are taught, as a matter of course, basic human biology, then we would be better prepared for life's knocks, that there would be less need for major mop-up operations later in life. This is not a plea for smiley faces everywhere, a Prozac nation too doped up to be arsed about anything, but a greater tolerance and understanding of the emotional fallout of trauma, and a recognition that therapy is not always self-indulgent quackery, but genuinely helpful. It is all too easy, when things are going well, to dismiss therapy as touchy-feely nonsense, to champion cool, rational thought. When things go spectacularly wrong, as they did for me, it is sometimes impossible to keep a cool head, go for the intellectual approach, ignore messy feelings. The effort is too much. Quite simply, it fucks you up.

Therapy, for me, has been an extraordinary and weird experience, but not dramatic. There's no movie script there, no moment of revelation. But life's rarely like that. I was completely traumatised by my cancer, but I was functioning. I had not, on the surface, gone under. I was, in basic Freudian terms, able to love and to work. But I was in a bad way – and now, most of the time, I'm not. Maybe this would have happened naturally, without the therapy, as I recovered and matured. But maybe not. I'm convinced not.

One unfortunate side-effect of this process has been that I can no longer believe in the narrative arc that is the basis of most features journalism. Stories open with a crisis – fat bottom, diagnosis of terminal illness – proceed apace to period of chaos, followed swiftly by journey to enlightenment and a nice happy ending. I always thought this arc was pretty suspect, cheap, a distortion of reality, but I used to think it was essentially harmless. Now I think it's cruel, depressing. I loathe reading these simplistic stories, particularly the cancer stories where I can see the gaping holes in the writer's neat narrative arc. As a freelance writer now, I try to resist writing them, too. It's hard though if you want to work for mainstream publications. Editors are obsessed with them. It has frequently been suggested to me that I ask interview subjects 'what they have learned', 'how they have changed', as if we were all capable of such feats and, even more optimistically, capable of articulating our achievements in bullet points. I was once asked by a magazine to get some extra quotes for an interview I'd done. The email outlined what information was required and suggested what the quotes would say. It's a small step away from making up stories.

Another unfortunate side-effect of therapy for me is that having learned to discern unhelpful patterns in my own behaviour, I see them more in other people. I have my behavioural tics but I am not unique. In my generation, they often seem to stem from a false sense of mastery of the universe. It is a modern phenomenon. How could it be otherwise? We have never been tested like our grandparents and parents. We have had no wars on the home front. Whatever we like to think, we have not had to struggle so much against sexism, notions of class. We are more affluent. And, despite the fact that we are reaping the rewards of a previous generation's hard work and vision, we somehow feel we are the powerful ones, invincible. We do not believe in unhappy endings. And so I was outraged, everyone I knew was outraged, when I was diagnosed with cancer and then discovered that I could not be cured. This was not supposed to happen. But we had hoodwinked ourselves. We are not masters of our own destiny. Terrible things do still happen.

The terrible aspect of cancer is, of course, its association with death, and one of the themes I have come back to over and over again in my therapy is the fear of death; mine and everybody else's. My experience has taught me that few people can bear to discuss death, my possible death. The fear is so great that it cannot, must not be discussed. Whenever I have tried, the subject is changed. Some people can listen for a while, then pass the buck, offering some quick fix – aromatherapy, yoga, crystals. Anything but connect. Those who do seem almost like another – I would say superior – species.

I am not obsessed with talking about death, but I have been forced to think about it. It is part of my life now. Elisabeth Kubler-Ross, who carried out ground-breaking work on the treatment of the terminally ill, found that the dying suffer when there is denial and that honesty is liberating. The trouble is, there is not much of it about. Language seems to fail us. Each death is seen as a tragedy, an affront, even when someone is quite old. Surely we can do better than that and surely the first step is to talk about death more openly.

We seem able to talk about sex more nowadays, money, religion, all the old taboos. But death still scares us witless. It's preposterous. I have come a long way in my thinking about death. I know that I do not want to be put on a ventilator or resuscitated – or resurrected as my grandmother described it – if I become seriously ill. I know that I would like to be buried in Brompton Cemetery although I do not know if that is possible. If not, maybe my ashes could be buried there and some sprinkled in the garden in Shropshire. I'm not so keen on that though because I worry that it would be difficult to think about selling the cottage if I'm in the garden. I would like the funeral service to be held at St Mary's in the Boltons. I would like flowers and I would like everyone to dress up, wear bright colours, wear hats. I would like lots of people to stand up and say nice things about me. I would, not surprisingly, like Lucian and Cosima to be swaddled with love. I would like Simon to find a new partner sooner rather than later. I would like all of them to grab at life, enjoy it, not forget me, but to remember me by making the most of their lives, to remember that it is possible to grieve and to live. These are not things that most 46-year-olds have thought about. Even so, I am not immune to the shock of death and dying. I am far from enlightened.

When I started writing this book in the summer of 2003, I had great plans for my new life as an author. I had already written a synopsis, so I had a map of the book. I made a schedule, so many words per week with an allowance for rewriting and additions. Instead of starting one Monday, I procrastinated until the Wednesday, but I managed to catch up with myself. Then life intervened.

First, it became apparent that my father was dying. He had been diagnosed with a brain tumour in 2001, but the tumour was accessible and he had surgery, followed by radiotherapy. He recovered quickly and, for a while, he was well. Then he started having what can only be described as turns. He fell over. He became confused. The tumour was back. He had surgery again, recovered quickly again, but just as quickly became ill again. He could not have any more radiotherapy – he'd had his quota – and chemotherapy wasn't effective on his kind of tumour. My mother became his nurse as he became ever weaker, eventually unable to walk. A stair lift was installed in their house, a special armchair was bought. A walking frame and wheelchair were delivered. All too soon, they became redundant as my father became bedridden and started sleeping more and more.

The expense was enormous from the outset. His first symptom – collapsing without warning into his soup one evening – was dismissed by his GP. He collapsed on a plane to Sicily and, during that holiday, spent an afternoon utterly confused, not knowing where he was. Back home, he was referred for heart tests. The waiting list was six to nine months, so my parents paid to jump the queue. There was nothing wrong with his heart and the specialist referred my father for neurological tests. The waiting list was again six to nine months, so my parents paid again. A tumour was discovered and emergency surgery scheduled. Their money had saved his life. Later, when they bought the stair lift and armchair, it was their money that enabled him to escape from the bedroom in which he had become imprisoned, to spend time downstairs, in the garden, and be taken to the day centre at the local hospice. My parents didn't resent this. My mother's reasoning was that my father had worked hard all his life – very hard, I would say – and deserved whatever they could afford from their savings. They were also socialists – we all are – but when push came to shove, it seemed to be their self-reliance, their prudence, those most Thatcherite of traits, that helped them.

The money issue was trivial though compared to the emotional shockwaves that went through the family. My father had always been so fit, so healthy – how could he be felled like this? He wasn't even 70. For me, there was the added confusion I felt about my father joining me in the cancer world. Our cancers were different. Did I know what he was going through or not? Did I have insider knowledge that would be helpful or not? I certainly knew nothing about brain cancer, but I knew much about the emotional impact of cancer. Occasionally we talked about this, but not often, and it felt topsy-turvy, unnatural, a daughter advising a father on how to deal with fear, discussing the merits of euthanasia. It seemed wrong that I had thought more about death than he had.

Sometimes this made me feel as though I was being melodramatic. When he had his first surgery, I went with my mother to the hospital and insisted we stay until he was called, defying the nurse who suggested we leave him to wait alone and thought that he would be 'fine'. I was incensed by her. We walked with him as he was wheeled into the operating theatre. After we had kissed him goodbye and he disappeared through the swing doors, I cried. For him and for myself. For the fact that this was only the slip road on to the motorway with a hard drive ahead and the destination vague, something which I had not been able to grasp at the time of my own surgery and was convinced my father had not grasped either.

It also felt odd because I was a survivor. When my father was first diagnosed, I knew the outlook was bleak, but his initial recovery was encouraging. Maybe he, too, would be a survivor. Then suddenly it became clear that he wouldn't be and I felt strange. I knew I was watching him. Is this how you die? Is this the best way to approach it? Is there any choice? Little things bothered me. There is no way a stair lift can be installed in a top-floor flat. More important issues – how to talk about death, how to support my parents appropriately – kept me awake at night. And the whole process undermined my confidence in what I was writing. How could survival be a problem when this was the alternative?

Then something else happened. It was July 2003. I was working at home and the phone rang. It was my sister Nellie. She was distressed. Her husband David had collapsed at work in London and she was on her way from Brighton to see him. He was at University College Hospital. I said I would meet her there. I jumped on the tube. It was hot and I ran, sweating, through the streets. I got there before her. She had told me to ask for the family room in casualty and I was taken there by a nurse. Waiting there was David's boss, Dennis. I asked him how David was. He said it didn't look good. I asked the nurse. She said she couldn't discuss anything until Nellie arrived. And then I realised he was dead. He was 49 and, we later found out, had had a heart attack. He had had no symptoms and had died while talking to a colleague. One minute he was standing by a desk, talking. The next he was on the floor, dead.

I had to wait nearly an hour for Nellie to arrive. The traffic was bad. She rang on her mobile to give us updates on her progress. When she arrived, she looked through the window in the door. She waved and smiled. And then I told her. I felt like I was destroying her life.

I still can't believe David is dead. It sometimes seems as though he has just gone on a long trip. I try to support Nellie. My mother sometimes says she thinks our family is jinxed. I don't. I just think we're a big family and this stuff happens. But the summer of 2003 was the worst I'd had since the summer I was diagnosed. Lucian and Cosima were distraught – they adored David – and I felt I was grieving not for David, but for Nellie and their marriage, which was one of the best I have ever seen, a beacon of hope in a world which can sometimes feel as though it is full of nasty, unkind marriages. And I felt even more tentative about this book. I was faced with another alternative to surviving and, again, there seemed to be no contest.

As the months rolled by and Nellie struggled with her grief, my father became more ill. But we were confused. The protocol was unclear. Who was in charge of his palliative treatment? Why did the GP never call and was he supposed to? How was my mother supposed to assess what was happening to my father? Was she entitled to help, and what kind of help? When should he go into the hospice? And why was my mother's friend told that her husband couldn't stay in the hospice because he was taking too long to die? Was there a timetable here? There was, in the jargon, no joined-up thinking. It was a vertical learning curve. When we are born, there's a system of midwives and health visitors and check-ups – not perfect but pretty slick. When we are dying, it seems, it's make-it-up-as-you-go-along time, each of us facing it as if we were the first. I recently heard Armistead Maupin talking on the radio about the extraordinary expertise that the gay community now has in dealing with death and dying because of the AIDS crisis, and I thought, someone should harness this, it's invaluable.

David had the kind of death that most people think they want, although not at 49. It was fast and, in theory, he knew very little about it. It must have hurt – someone told me that it must have been like being shot – but not for long. He suffered none of the indignities of old age or illness. There was no harrowing treatment, no waiting to die, no watching the pain on Nellie's face. There were no worries about what would happen to her without him. There was no anger about what he might miss. But there was also no time to say goodbye. It was, I think, the best and worst of deaths. My father had time to sort out his affairs, to mull over his life, to tell us all how much he loved us, but he also had to face two lots of brain surgery, the slow and gradual loss of his independence, the guilt of being a burden to my mother who lovingly nursed him until the end, enabling him to die where he wanted to, at home with her. They had been together for 50 years, entirely devoted to each other.

So there I was, as I started writing, surrounded by death, and I kept hearing that broken record: this was not supposed to happen. This was not fair. I tried to resist listening to it. I knew it was nonsense. These deaths were sad, the saddest I have ever experienced, but not outrageous. And there was another problem. I was alive, very much alive, and trying to write about the difficulties of not being dead, of surviving. How could I possibly do that in such circumstances? How selfish and self-indulgent would that seem? And then it clicked. Nothing had changed. My questions were answering themselves. These deaths were having the same effect on me as everything else I had struggled with since my diagnosis, and my conclusion would be no different. The reason it is so difficult to survive – and to write about surviving – is because everyone, including me, knows it could be worse. *I am so lucky to survive* is the general gist of it. You must leap out of bed every morning, jumping for joy! And it's not like that, actually.

6

Praise You

When I talk about my recovery from being ill, my attempt at surviving cancer with some dignity, I most often talk about my psychological state, whereas it is, of course, my physical state that gave rise to my psychological state. My relationship with my body is so complex though that I cannot separate the two states. Other people do not share this ambivalence. They have 'views'. I was bombarded with them when I had chemotherapy.

Until then, nobody had ever mentioned that I bore even the slightest resemblance to Demi Moore, the American actress who first made waves appearing pregnant and naked on the cover of *Vanity Fair* magazine. But suddenly, we seemed to have an awful lot in common. 'Don't worry,' friends would say whenever the subject of my impending baldness came up. 'You'll look great. Look at Demi Moore.' It wasn't that they were advocating I strip off for a magazine, but rather that I take comfort from the fact that, at the time, she had shaved her head for a role. Two other glamorous baldies were also forced on me as role models: another actress – Sigourney Weaver, the *Alien 3* version – and the singer Sinead O'Connor. I felt depressed. Even though the raw material was the best – maybe a nine or a ten – and they were plastered with clever make-up, these women still looked grim to me. I would, I knew, as a mere five, look even worse with no hair. And I did. But – and this is a big but – by the time I went completely bald, I didn't really care. I didn't like it, but I didn't hate it either.

At first, I was appalled by the thought of having no hair. It didn't help that the hospital couldn't tell me how quickly it would fall out as everyone reacts differently to chemotherapy. All I knew was that during the three months of chemo in outpatients, in order to conserve my hair, I would wear a cool cap, a rather tame description for what was, back then, an extremely heavy helmet which was supposed to chill the hair follicles and prevent chemicals penetrating, slowing down hair loss in some patients. Note the 'some'. During the stem cell transplant, the rest of my hair would fall out – definitely. There would be no cool caps on offer then and the implication was that being bald would be the least of my problems.

The chemo nurse suggested I have my thick shoulder-length hair cut short – as short as possible – before treatment started so that any hair loss would be less noticeable and therefore, her reasoning went, less traumatic. I did as I was told and went to see the hairdresser Trevor Sorbie who has his own salon in the West End. This rather grand appointment was arranged by a colleague who knew him. She had explained to him why I needed this haircut.

I have had, like everyone else, thousands of haircuts in my life, some good, some that made me agoraphobic. And there has always been a slight tension about the process. Our hair is one of the few aspects of our appearance that can be changed easily and we all have ludicrous expectations of its ability to transform us. This haircut felt different though. I didn't feel tense. I felt melancholic. It wasn't so much the style that mattered but why I was having it done. The process felt ritualistic and the image that kept coming into my mind was of the way bodies are prepared for burial. There was also some notion floating around in my head about Samson and loss of potency.

Trevor was kind and knew a lot about hair loss, which normalised the situation for me. Some people have this knack and it's a gift. He didn't faff around talking about Demi Moore, he just discussed my hair and what was going to happen to it. And he made it fun. When I said that I wanted to go really short, he told me that it was a treat for him to chop, really chop, into a head of thick, long hair. And he gave me such an excellent haircut that, for a couple of weeks, I forgot about the hair issue.

Then after only two doses of chemo, to my absolute horror, my hair started to fall out. I woke up one morning to find the pillow covered in hair and when I touched my head handfuls came out. I was plunged into depression. It felt like the last straw, perhaps another last straw, humiliating, undignified. The next time I washed my hair – which I'd been told to do gently and with baby shampoo – so much fell out that I became hysterical. I rang Simon at work and asked him to come home. This probably sounds like an over-reaction and, even at the time, I felt it was. But I couldn't help myself and I gradually realised that my reaction had very little to do with vanity – although it was an element – and everything to do with denial. Up until then, I had been able to hide the damage that my cancer had wreaked on my body – if you'd seen me in the street, you would not have known that I had cancer – but there was no hiding the hair loss and therefore no hiding my cancer from the world, and so, of course, myself. I was becoming a marked woman, a woman with cancer. The hair loss acted like a battering ram, slowly but surely denting my armour of denial which was already in a bad way from the other side-effects of the chemotherapy.

I tried to be practical. I wasted hours in front of the mirror arranging scarves round my head in an attempt to look like Princess Caroline when she lost her hair. But no, I looked like Mrs Mop or one of those deranged, anorexic ballet teachers. I then went in search of a hat. It was the height of summer and all I could find were wedding hats or big beach hats, which looked absurd and, even if I had forced myself to wear them, were usually made of straw and too scratchy for my vulnerable scalp. I was about to give up when, much to my amazement, I found a little black velvet skullcap at Prada. I told the baffled assistant that I had to try it on in the changing room and, behind closed doors, experimented to see what it would look like with no hair showing at all. A bit odd, I decided, a bit medieval, but it would do.

In fact, I had panicked early. My hair didn't fall out suddenly. It just got thinner and thinner and, as I had very thick hair, even half a head of hair left me looking vaguely normal before the stem cell treatment. But there was one problem I still hadn't resolved: the wig. From the start, the hospital had said that I ought to get a wig and choose one before I went bald so that I could get a good copy of my normal colour and style. Trevor had also said he would help me choose one and adapt it, if necessary. But however much I tried, I could not imagine myself wearing a wig. I was hardly in the mood for making fashion statements à la Sinead, but I was convinced that I would look and feel like a transvestite in a wig. The pageboy wig that the MP Mo Mowlam was wearing at the time, after her much-publicised treatment for a brain tumour, didn't help. I am far from the cutting edge of fashion, but a pageboy in 1997? I couldn't face it. The hospital arranged for a brochure and hair samples to be sent to my home. I didn't know whether to laugh or cry when they arrived. What to choose from? Farrah Fawcett during her *Charlie's Angels* period? Thelma's brushed-forward helmet in *The Likely Lads*? All in shimmering synthetic. I threw the lot in the bin. One alternative was a hand-made job, a mere £1,500. Forget it.

Luckily, Simon also thought a wig was a ridiculous idea. But there was subtle pressure from some friends. One went as far as to suggest that I'd be housebound if I didn't get a wig, but most just told me that I'd come round to the idea. They probably didn't mean to be patronising but, at this point, I started to get annoyed. Didn't I have more important things to worry about? If I'd broken my leg, would the hospital have handed me a brown envelope containing a catalogue of long skirts? Do men get sent the wig brochure? I doubt it very much. Then the letter from Katy arrived, explaining that she'd ordered one and hated it so much that she'd never worn it. That did it. If she could get by with a few hats, then so could I. Later, I discovered that Shirley, too, had ordered and discarded a wig. It looked odd, she said, and was unbearably itchy. Francine had two wigs, one sensible, like her own short brown hair, the other blonde, Barbie-style, an option I never thought of and wish I had. It was a wasted opportunity.

I went into hospital for the stem cell transplant in mid-October armed with my Prada hat for indoors, and a cheapo

fake-fur number from Accessorize for outside. I was determined to be pragmatic and when my hair started falling out in
clumps, it so got on my nerves – it was like having a cat in the
bed – that I asked for my head to be shaved. As the handsome
young Norwegian nurse propped me up on a chair and set to
work with the clippers, I asked him whether he'd done this
before. 'Oh yes,' he said confidently. 'On a sheep.' And that was
that. I was bald. It had finally happened and I didn't shed a
single tear. I looked appalling though. On the rare occasions
when I looked in the mirror, I felt as if I was looking at someone
else. I tried to merge the person I felt I was with the person in
the mirror and I couldn't. Friends said I was lucky that I had
such good bones, that the shape of my head was so neat, but it
was all rubbish. I looked like an inmate of a concentration camp.
I was not only bald, but skinny, pale and hunched from the
physical and emotional sledgehammer of the treatment. My
eyelashes had thinned, my eyebrows were patchy. My face
lacked all definition. In short, I looked terrible. The only benefit
was that the hair on my legs and in my armpits fell out, too, so I
didn't have to shave. Oddly my pubic hair wasn't affected. It
was not the first time I had pondered the absurdity of women's
relationship with their hair.

Back home, Lucian was not won over by my fabulous
cheekbones. He had been told that I would lose my hair, but the
first time he saw me bald, he screamed, 'You look horrible. You
look like an old builder.' I'm not sure what an old builder looks
like, but it's obviously not great and I had to draw on every
ounce of maturity to say, 'Oh, don't worry, it will grow back
soon.' Although I was upset to see him so upset, I was also
relieved. Other people's pussy-footing around was exhausting.

I knew they were just being nice to me, which made me feel patronised, separate. Lucian was engaging with me as he always did, on the level, as a normal person with, well, standards, not someone who would go around looking like crap and not notice. I had to promise that I would not go to his school, and would wear a hat if anyone came to the house. Cosima was more bemused than angry but pretty keen that I keep a hat on.

They calmed down after a few days. Lucian had made me a Welcome Home card depicting me bald and smiling, and said that, really, I looked the same but without hair, and Cosima kindly lent me a few of her dressing-up hats. But at bedtime, they would both say rather plaintively that they preferred me 'like this', pointing at the photographs of me with long hair that they'd stuck on their bedheads when I was in hospital. What they preferred, of course, was the mother I was before I was ill, the mother they used to have, the more reliable one. It wasn't just the hair that was different to them. I was. And both, of course, for the worse.

I stuck to the two-hat routine and found that in Shropshire, where there is no central heating, I often needed to wear a hat in bed, too. You get very cold without hair. I took to wearing make-up more often than not – not my usual mode – and I found that, as having no hair made me look, let's face it, a bit butch, I had to be careful what I wore. Loose shirts and tailored jackets were out. I looked better in soft, fitted clothes. As my confidence grew, I gradually stopped wearing a hat indoors but I had to harden myself to the sight of visitors trying oh-so-hard to keep their cool when they saw me bald for the first time. In fact, I got to hate this initial reaction so much that when people came to visit, as soon as I had buzzed them in, I would shout down the hallway, 'Don't forget I'm bald.' As time went on, there were fewer cracks about Demi Moore. More often I was simply reassured: 'Don't worry, it'll grow back in no time.' And from my friend, Deirdre, when she took me out for a posh lunch at the Savoy and I briefly removed my hat to show her how bald I was, 'very *Gulag Archipelago*, darling'.

It took a few months before I had any noticeable hair and it was only then that I started taking off my hat in public. People stared, but I was feeling stronger by then and could cope with a few funny looks – although I didn't enjoy the 'Christ Almighty' comment I got from a passing male colleague when I first went back to work. On a good day I could just about convince myself that I looked like someone with a rather bad haircut and on a bad day, well, I resigned myself to the fact that I looked like I'd escaped from the set of *Prisoner: Cell Block H*, and steered clear of mirrors and shop windows. As for the children, Lucian's main worry was that, as my hair grew, I would somehow metamorphose into a woman with long blonde hair, high heels and a tight dress. Barbie, I suppose. The logic was impeccable. I have never, since my teens, worn high heels and rarely tight dresses, but if I could change once, he probably reasoned, it was entirely possible that I could change again.

Now my hair is exactly the same as it used to be, possibly slightly thinner, but that may be due to age rather than the treatment. But when it first started to grow back, it was curly, really curly. It felt springy, like a camomile lawn. My hair had never been curly, not even as a baby, so it was fascinating. The same thing happened to Shirley and I learned that sometimes, after chemo, hair can grow back a different colour – grey, or the colour it was before it went grey. My eyelashes also grew back thick and curly, very different. At the same time, I started growing new fingernails over my old ones which looked disgusting. It was as if my body was starting all over again with renewed vigour. Then, slowly and almost imperceptibly, everything went back to normal. My hair got straighter, my eyelashes spindlier.

Well, everything visible to that stranger in the street went back to normal. I had survived looking weird and I was glad that I hadn't got a wig. Obviously it helped that I was bald in the winter when hats are more acceptable and that my baldness was short-term – alopecia and long-term chemo pose different problems. But it really wasn't so bad having no hair and probably not as bad as wearing a rather unconvincing, itchy wig. Nobody took much notice after an initial gawp and, as anyone who's gone through the misery of cancer treatment knows, you soon stop caring what you look like. Not totally, but enough to get you through. And, as Simon said rather enviously during one of my bad no-hair days, 'At least yours will grow back.'

Breasts don't grow back, of course, and one of the most interesting things about breast cancer is that, while the general public thinks that losing a breast is a tragedy and the main body issue for women, I have never met anyone who has had a mastectomy who really gives a damn. Breasts are symbolic in our culture – of sexuality and nurturing, of women's supposed essence – and it is therefore presumed that the loss of a breast is devastating in a way that the loss of, say, an ear is not. For many women, it isn't.

For me, once I knew that I was going to have a mastectomy, I wanted it done quickly. I wanted to be rid of my cancer. The devastation was about the cancer, not the breast I was going to lose. I was relieved that I had the type of cancer that could be felt, by me and by my doctors. Other cancers are often much more advanced before they can be detected and then only by medical tests, rather than your own hands. You can't examine your ovaries or colon in the way that you can examine your breasts. I was *relieved* that my breast could be cut off. You can't cut out your entire brain or liver. And I was relieved that, although I would be scarred, those scars wouldn't be visible when I was dressed. Facial disfigurement or the amputation of a limb is much more of a challenge. And I was relieved that my lack of breast and the scars would not prevent me from doing anything. I wasn't going to lose my ability to walk, speak, to eat normally, or any of the many other possible consequences of cancer surgery. So I didn't, as many presume, feel less of a woman. That was completely beside the point. I felt lucky.

My reconstruction is good, but no reconstruction is perfect. My breasts are asymmetrical because I should really have my other breast enhanced – most women who have reconstructions need to have the other breast enhanced, reduced or lifted, as it's nigh on impossible to get a perfect match, particularly when you are over 30 and have had children. Reconstructed breasts don't tend to have nipples either. I've been told that I can have one made and that this can be 'done' when I have that other breast enhanced. I've had enough surgery for now though. I'm really not convinced about fake nipples – they sound rubbery to me –

and I'm happy to wear a pad on my left-hand side to even things up. It's a compromise, but not one that I think about much.

I'm not self-conscious about my body at home. Simon has never got down on his knees and kissed my scars, slushy-novel style. He's just accepting. 'I think we're beyond that,' he said when I told him I felt I looked a mess. I've never hidden anything from the children. The pad I wear is made of silicone and they are fascinated by it. Lucian was once asking me about it but couldn't remember what it was called – prosthesis is not a terribly child-friendly word – and decided it was my spare brain. I like that. But I don't like, and avoid, communal changing rooms. I won't go for a massage unless I feel very comfortable with the masseuse. I don't much like wearing a swimming costume. I've got a nice enough costume that covers and supports my complicated breasts, and conceals the long scar which runs from the middle of my back to underneath my breast, but I don't feel completely confident in it. And although I've probably not enjoyed wearing a swimming costume since my pert and skinny twenties, the awkwardness I feel now is different. Before, I was aware that I was off-the-mark in the supermodel standards of beauty, but then so is most of the population. I was also, like most women with children, resigned to the idea of bodily wear and tear, flab and stretch marks. But now I was in a minority of the disfigured. It was hard to adjust.

Immediately after my mastectomy I was told to get myself a substantial, supportive bra and that I should wear it day and night until told otherwise. I was worried about where I would find one as I had no idea what size I was any more. I went to Rigby & Peller, next to Harrods, where I had been once before. They were wonderful. It's a tiny shop that sells just underwear and some swimwear. You walk in and queue up for a fitting, waiting on little gold chairs. When it's your turn, you are taken into a changing room and assessed – visually, not with tape measures – and are then brought bra after bra to try on until you find one that's right. I was nervous and self-conscious as I undressed, but the assistant was so matter-of-fact that I soon relaxed. We've seen it all before, she said. This looks good. You should see some of them, she said. Boob-jobs up near their shoulders, lopsided, lumpy. We sort them all out. This is no problem. I've never gone anywhere else for bras since.

It's a palaver though and I could do without it. I could also do without the reaction of most men to the news that I have had breast cancer. As I say the words, their eyes drift south, some-times subtly, sometimes obviously, to my breasts. What are they looking for? A horror show? A show-and-tell? It's fantastically irritating. Women, apart from those insanely competitive types, never do it. Sometimes I wish I didn't care what I looked like at all but I can't and don't identify with those women who choose to be visibly one-breasted. When I read Audre Lorde's account of her breast cancer, of her vision of a horde of amazons marching on the White House demanding an end to the scourge, I mentally cheered her on. But I wasn't willing to take up the challenge. When I met the yoga teacher, Julie Friedeberger, who is also one-breasted, I cheered her on, too. But I didn't for a second regret my decision to have a reconstruction and my continuing attempts to look normal.

I have been a feminist all my life and I've been on many marches. I belonged to a feminist book and discussion group throughout my twenties. I've danced round bonfires at Greenham Common. I've read the set texts and I know that women are oppressed by impossible and ever-changing standards of beauty, and waste enormous amounts of energy and money trying to live up to them. I know that, in an ideal world, women would not need to have reconstructions and wear prostheses. And although I had the energy to deal with being bald, somehow I don't have the energy to make a stand about this issue. There's denial in there somewhere but it's also something to do with my thoughts about recovery. I think that even in my foggy mental state back when I was making treatment decisions, I knew that I would be making compromises. The wig question was containable. The one-breast question would, if I was lucky, go on and on and on. I needed to pace myself.

I do have some physical problems. Nobody gets off scot-free with cancer treatment. But they impinge on me very little at the moment – I choose not to think about the long-term effects of my treatment because I have such a tentative grasp of the concept of long-term. I really can't tell if my immune system has been affected. I did get shingles a couple of years after my treatment, which was truly appalling. I do seem to get ill more than before I was diagnosed, but it may be an age thing. I don't know. I may just be more neurotic. One irritation I am aware of is that my digestion is not as good as it used to be. Another is that I have to keep my shoulder and back supple. They stiffen up remarkably quickly. My nerves and muscles took a big hit in surgery. I was, up to a point, prepared for this. I also knew about lymphoedema, the condition where a limb – in my case my right arm where my lymph nodes were removed – can swell horribly and irreversibly after surgery. So, immediately after my mastectomy, I did a boring series of exercises day after day, often a couple of times a day, and applied vitamin E oil to the scars. I soon gave up the oily mess but still do a version of the exercises. They work. Later when I developed back problems – I slipped a disc – an osteopath told me that I was slightly twisted from the surgery. A more relevant factor, I think, is that the whole experience made me so tense that my back became a disaster waiting to happen. All I do know for sure is that if I don't exercise, my shoulder and chest become uncomfortably tight and, if I do nothing about it, the rest of my back seizes up. It's tedious, but at least I can do something to help myself.

I have also found yoga helpful. I had been to classes when I was pregnant with Cosima, but as soon as she was born, I'd found them dull, dull, dull. Over the years, I tried a few other classes, which weren't dull but were too hard, too demanding, too much balancing on one leg. But after my back went, I tried again. And I loved it. The reason was simple: I found the right teacher, Julie Friedeberger. I had read about her class at the Yoga Therapy Centre in London in a now-defunct magazine called *Bare* and realised that the centre was five minutes from where I was working at the time. It was a class for people with cancer and was gentle. We didn't talk about cancer, but there was a warm feeling of support and understanding in the class, facilitated by Julie's own experience of breast cancer. Some people were, like me, in post-treatment limbo, some were having chemo, some were dealing with recurrences and some were dying. The class was a time-out for us all. When I changed job, I found a class nearer home at a local adult education centre which I still attend. I lucked out again with the teacher, Ruby Lawson, who is also gentle and unfailingly patient with people like me who still find the sun salutation a serious challenge.

Apart from the physical benefits, the reason that I have stuck with yoga is that it has helped me to be patient, to stay, if only briefly, in the present, not fret about the past or future, that impossible task that so many low-grade self-help books throw at us, because yoga is as much a psychological exercise as it is physical. When you concentrate on your breathing, standing on one leg, whatever, you can't think about anything else – it's impossible – and that's a release, a holiday for the mind. And these time-outs from minor and major worries have, in turn, given me a taste for the pleasures of the journey, rather than the arrival, a way of looking at life which has often been suggested to me but which I find difficult to embrace, being by nature an arrivals kind of person, goal-orientated. It doesn't spill over into the rest of my life much, but a little, enough to make a difference sometimes, to lower my anxiety levels. When I can't sleep, for example, I practise my yoga breathing, concentrate on it so hard that my mind empties and, if my mind won't empty, I think about how my life is *right now*, this minute. I think about how, right now, this minute, I am safe in bed with Simon next to me, I am not ill, my children are fine. Tomorrow? Who knows. Right now, everything is fine.

One of the things I never worry about though is that I am now infertile. It is, for me, one of the perks of having cancer. When I started chemo, I was told that my periods would probably stop and that when I had the stem cell transplant, my ovaries might destroyed. As, at 39, I was probably approaching the menopause anyway and would be taking tamoxifen for five years, Professor Coombes thought my periods would never come back – with younger women they sometimes do after standard chemo. He was right and I am thrilled. I was lucky, I know. I had two children and didn't want any more. Other women are just starting out on motherhood, have had a first child and want another when they are diagnosed. Other women, who had thought that they would have children later, suddenly find out that there might not be a later and if there is, it won't include children.

The technology is there, after a fashion, to help these women – removing eggs pre-chemo, saving them, etc. – but it's far from infallible, so some women make the decision to delay treatment to try for a baby. These women terrify me. If they are in their late thirties, early forties, they sometimes decide not to have chemo at all. If they are younger, they might have the chemo, but not take the tamoxifen. Every time I hear about these women, I want to shout, no, no, no. I don't, of course. They have the right to choose. But all too often I hear later that their cancer has come back, quickly. Some of these women then die, unnecessarily I believe. Maybe their cancer would have come back anyway. But maybe it wouldn't. Or at least not as quickly. These women say that their lives aren't worth living if they can't have a baby and I have to believe them. But I also feel angry that they aren't selfish enough to put their own health first, and that we live in a society where it is still considered selfish or odd not to have children.

My challenge was easier, to handle the menopause at 40. It was difficult though to differentiate between menopausal symptoms and the side-effects of the tamoxifen itself. Most women seem to experience some sort of vaginal discharge on tamoxifen. I did, and it was irritating but hardly life-threatening. Some women say they put on weight, too. I'm not convinced. I did put on weight, but it was because I exercised less and ate more for a while, treating myself after nearly starving to death during the stem cell transplant. And I liked being heavier. Being skinny has become synonymous with illness to me in much the same way, I suppose, that it did for the gay community when AIDS started spreading, although I did not react by going in for body-building, just being lazier. Weight fluctuation unnerves me, too. Every January I had to tell myself that when I went back to normal eating after Christmas, I was just losing podge. It wasn't a sign of my cancer returning.

The most onerous part of my early menopause was the hot flushes, five years of them. At first they seemed to be more or less continuous, making me feel a berk in the day and keeping me awake at night. A hot flush works like this: suddenly and without any warning, you feel absolutely boiling hot. If you are lucky, you glisten. If not, you are drenched in sweat. I was somewhere in the middle. When it happened I felt compelled to rip off as many clothes as was decent. By day, I wore twinsets – sleeveless tops with matching cardigans which I never buttoned – so that I could take off the top layer quickly and modestly. At night, I would throw off the duvet. Seconds later, I would be shivering as my body compensated for the rise in temperature, so it was back on with the cardigan or duvet. And, of course, my face would be bright red throughout. It was excruciatingly embarrassing because it made me look as though I was, well, embarrassed about something, not coping, flipping out, the complete opposite of the image I tried to project at work. In the end, I resorted to explaining to people what was happening to me. Women tended to sympathise. Men looked uncomfortable.

Over the years, the hot flushes became less dramatic and less frequent, and a couple of months after I stopped taking tamoxifen, they more or less stopped, coincidentally the time when many of my older friends were starting to experience peri- or actual menopausal symptoms. They were full of the horrors of disturbed nights, damp clothes, sensitive skin. When I reminded them that I had already had the menopause, they gave me advice about HRT and other, what they called natural, remedies. I reminded them that it wasn't exactly advisable to go mucking around with my hormones and I didn't think they should either. All this would pass, I explained. It wasn't so bad. This was supposed to happen. They wouldn't have it though and threw away their money on creams and pills. They felt their bodies had betrayed them and this I understood.

I could, on some level, absorb all the physical degradations of my treatment. What I couldn't bear was the way my body had let me down. My diagnosis destroyed my trust in my body. Up until then, I felt it had stood by me. It had been healthy. It had supported me through years of working long, long hours in newspaper offices and through two pregnancies and births in my thirties. It had fuctioned well, so I thought. It was my ally. I wasn't sickly. I got pregnant easily. I gave birth easily. I went back to work easily-ish. And then, out of the blue, catastrophe. I was not ill. I had no symptoms. I found a lump. I had cancer. I could die. My body became the enemy and I felt that it had crept up on me in the night.

For a while, I struggled to find a reason why I had developed breast cancer. I raked over my medical history for clues. My periods started when I was 13, hardly early, and I had Lucian when I was 33, not that late for a first child. I'd breastfed both my children. I'd taken the pill for a couple of years in my late teens and twenties, then again for under a year just before I was diagnosed. I'd had mastitis while breastfeeding. I'd had a large mole removed from my right breast. Did any of this mean anything? I'd never had a particularly high-fat diet and there didn't seem to be any breast cancer in our family medical history. It didn't add up to much. I obsessed over how I might have harmed myself. Was I too buttoned up? Was I one of those crazy Type A personalities? Had my work been too stressful? It was absurd – all sorts of people get cancer. I knew this was ridiculous, but it was hard to stop myself being seduced into self-blame when there seemed no other plausible causes.

I asked my doctors what they thought. They said they didn't know. One suggested that although the statistics suggested that a tiny minority of breast cancers are genetically determined, perhaps many more were but we hadn't identified the genes yet. He said I shouldn't give myself a hard time about my cancer. I shouldn't conclude that I had developed cancer because of something I had done to myself. Plenty of people had stressful jobs, he said. Some dropped dead when they retired. Everyone reacts differently to stress and nobody could say what would have happened to me if I had not had these jobs. Maybe I would have been more stressed by the frustration, he suggested. He also said that there were hormones everywhere in the environment which may or may not have affected me. Maybe I had a susceptibility to getting cancer. Maybe something came along in my life that then triggered it, the straw that broke the camel's back. Maybe not. In other words, there were no easy answers. After a couple of months, I stopped thinking about why I had cancer. I decided it was bad luck.

The trouble with this conclusion is that it makes me feel helpless. I did have the most phenomenal amount of cancer treatment, of course, but there's nothing for me to do now, so I'm left simply mistrusting my body. I am suspicious of it. I can't read it. If I didn't notice that I had cancer until it had spread to my lymph nodes, I reason, how on earth am I supposed to know what my body is up to now? All I know is that I need to be vigilant. What would reassure me is to have a total body scan every day, preferably by one of those new wow-you-can-see-everything scanners. That isn't an option surprisingly. When I came back from a trip to New York, I asked Professor Coombes about the treatment for breast cancer that some of the women I'd met there had had. It seemed that, in America, they were giving as first-line treatment the kind of stuff reserved for advanced breast cancer here. Should I have been given this treatment, I demanded to know? He was happy with the treatment I'd been given, he said. By then, I think he was used to my anxieties.

For a while, after my treatment finished, I became hypochondriac where I used to be robust. I raced back to the hospital on a number of occasions. Once, I developed a wheeze. Asthma is in my family and I am allergic to dogs and horses. The last time I had an attack was in my twenties, but I had been told to look out for breathlessness that did not go away, a sign that the cancer had spread to my lungs. I rang Professor Coombes' office, and was told to go in straight away. I had a chest X-ray. Afterwards, as I sat waiting to be told that the X-ray had taken, a technician came out and called me back in. I thought I would collapse. We can see something, he said. My legs started to buckle. But we wanted to ask you about it, he said. I looked. There was a bright white dot on the X-ray. It was the valve from my reconstruction. I laughed, after a fashion, an hysterical, desperate sort of laugh. I was given the X-ray and took it round to Professor Coombes. He said there was nothing there. If it was him, he said, he'd be more than happy with this X-ray. I felt foolish. I went home and slept, drained. The wheezing stopped.

Another time, a weekend, a lump came up under my left arm. Time stood still until I got on the phone. I could see Professor Coombes on the Tuesday morning. I became a zombie. Then, on the Monday evening, the lump disappeared. When I arrived at the hospital, I found Professor Coombes waiting for me in his office. Mr Sinnett was down the hall waiting for me, too. I was examined. They were baffled. I felt foolish. I went straight to bed when I got home and slept.

Another time, I had severe backache. I had been told to look out for aches and pains that did not go away, a sign that the cancer had spread to my bones. This time, I was about to have a check-up with Mr Sinnett. It was, for a change, at Charing Cross rather than at the Cromwell where I usually saw him. He said I should have a bone scan. I went upstairs to the unit. They said they were not sure they had enough supplies for the glow-in-the-dark injection I needed – it has to be ordered specially. I insisted, in an unattractive way, that I had to have the scan. Now. They found the stuff, I was injected. After the scan, I was told to make an appointment with Mr Sinnett to get the results. I said I wanted them. Now. They said that wasn't how it worked. I said I wasn't leaving until I got them. The head of the unit came in and said the protocol was that Mr Sinnett would tell me the results. I said that I knew he had looked at the scan, knew what was on it and I wanted the results. He went away for a while and then I was called into his office. He said he had spoken to Uncle Dudley and that he had been given permission to give me the results. So they're clear, I said. As far as we can see, he said. Outside in the corridor, I burst into tears. I went home and the backache disappeared. I still don't know if I'm more shocked by my own behaviour or the patronising Uncle Dudley comment.

Despite all evidence pointing to the fact that I was a serious hypochondriac and highly suggestible, at no point did anyone at the hospital tell me that I was wasting their time. In fact, I was always told that I had done the right thing. You never knew. I certainly never knew. I couldn't read my body. I was baffled by its behaviour and baffled by the thought that maybe I was *creating* these symptoms. When I came off tamoxifen, I started having migraines. Was this a physical reaction to stopping the drug? Was it a psychological reaction to having a crutch taken away? Was there something more sinister wrong with me or was I just having migraines? I was bewildered by the various mind–body permutations, floored by them. Other forms of bewilderment have made me panicky and rude. Once, when I went to Charing Cross for another chest X-ray, I surpassed myself. I was back at work by then and as there were no appointments for X-rays, I rang ahead to find out when the unit was quietest so that I could be seen quickly. The system is that you turn up, take a ticket like you do at the supermarket deli, and wait for your number to be called. You can wait for hours. They said it was less busy after 4pm. Then, when I arrived, I was told that I couldn't be seen because they only saw in-patients after 4pm.

There were four people hanging round the reception desk. The waiting area was deserted. I said I wasn't leaving until I got my X-ray. They stared at me. I stared back. Eventually one of them asked me if I'd been to the hospital before. I said I had, quite a few times actually, because I had been treated for cancer there. One of the women sighed and said, okay then, I'll do it. She walked round to my side of the desk, led me through the empty waiting room and into the X-ray room. I cried when I got home.

I'm still bolshie. When a registrar appeared at one of my check-ups instead of Professor Coombes, I told him that I didn't want to talk to him. I told him that I was sure he was brilliant, but I wanted to see Professor Coombes. He was polite and made another appointment for me. When I agreed to participate in the bone marrow trial, I complained about the trainees who occasionally carried out the procedure. Their tentativeness made it hurt more. One of these trainees said that she understood my reaction. But I never used to be like this, I said. You didn't know before, she said. You didn't know what real illness and pain felt like, and now you know, you're frightened of it.

I think terrified is a better word. Before I was diagnosed, I didn't know about the myriad ways in which my body could go wrong and could be treated. The surgery, the chemotherapy and, most horribly, the stem cell transplant took away my innocence. It has turned me into Little Miss Weedy. A bad headache has me thinking about brain tumours, racing for the painkillers where once I would have presumed I would sleep it off. When I slipped a disc and had an MRI, I was scared there was a tumour on my spine. The consultant obviously thought there might be, too, because when I got the results he was very careful to tell me not only which disc was affected but that there was 'nothing else to worry about', and the information was passed on to Mr Sinnett. I thought he handled the situation well. Often I don't.

When I suffered from severe neckache in 2002, I went along to my GP who said I should have an X-ray. He suggested I go immediately. On the form he gave me to take with me, it stated that I had had breast cancer. There were about 10 people before me and I watched them disappearing for their X-ray, reappearing and waiting to find out if it had taken and then being told that the results would be with their GP in around a week. When it came to me, I was told that I should make an appointment with my GP for the results as soon as possible, that they would be faxed through that afternoon. I flipped. There was obviously something on the X-ray. Cancer of the neck? Was there such a thing? I asked the technician what he could see. He couldn't tell me, he said. My GP would tell me.

At home, I went into a funk and Simon got on the phone, first to the GP who didn't seem too concerned and then on to Professor Coombes' office. They were concerned. Within the hour, the GP had rung back explaining that everything was fine and that he had suddenly realised why I was so worried, and the hospital had rung saying they had had the results faxed over and everything was fine. Just wear and tear, they said, and they thought that, given my medical history, I would feel better if I got the results quickly. The trouble is that quickly now means immediately for me, not just soon, otherwise the anxiety is unbearable. When I hear of people waiting weeks and months for tests and results, I am infuriated. The suffering it causes is appalling and why, oh why, does it take so long for results to be sent to a GP or consultant? I know that the technician who carries out the tests knows the results and I know that they have to be checked by a consultant, but surely this can happen faster, at least with scans and X-rays. Once when I had a bone scan, I asked the technician if everything was okay. I kept the question vague to see what would happen. He answered one of the possible questions I had asked, that, yes, the scan was technically fine. The consultant would be able to read it. Then, because he knew what I was really asking, he asked me if I wanted to look at it. I said I didn't know how to read a scan but I knew that he was telling me, in the only way that he could, that there was nothing suspicious on it. I was so grateful.

The experience with my neck was ghastly, though. I was in excruciating pain and I was in shock. That afternoon, we drove to Lucian's school for a carol concert in the chapel. He is in the choir and it was beautiful. Tears rolled down my face for most of it. I was alive. My cancer had not come back. I kept trying to imagine what I would be feeling if it had. And I was angry. Back in 1998 when my treatment had finished, Professor Coombes had told me that I should tell him if I had any symptoms I was worried about. He said that there was no point going to my GP. I had done as I was told, and then I hadn't. There I was in 2002 trying to be normal, trying to treat a neckache as a neckache, and I paid and paid for it. Simon brought up the subject first, saying never again, never again. You must go to Professor Coombes if you are worried about anything. But, but . . . I said. But he was right.

There's a book on my shelves called *Our Bodies, Ourselves*. It's one of those women-centred health books. It's very good. I used to refer to it frequently. I don't now. I hate the title. It reminds me of a time when I felt I could make choices about my body. It was probably an illusion because this feeling was never seriously tested. But it was a comforting illusion and I miss it. My relationship with my body is uneasy now. I watch it carefully, not really knowing what I am looking for, and when I find something, I'm not sure how to react. I always seem to get it wrong. And yet, and yet . . . it hasn't let me down totally yet. How do you cross all your fingers and toes?

7

Young Americans

It is one of the great ironies of my attitude to having cancer that, just as I thought I had settled on a way of dealing with it – quietly trying to have an ordinary life, doing my job, seeing Mrs Witham – I found myself contemplating one of those great life changes, one of those changes that I was convinced was the last thing I needed. I was thinking of giving up journalism and working for a cancer charity. There I was, on the brink of switching from being one cliché – the tragic young woman with breast cancer – to another, the woman who has suffered and is driven to give back, who has discovered what really matters. The reality was a little less romantic and dramatic, but still unnerving.

For a start, my first year back at work had been confusing. I had gone back in the February and, after a couple of months, my boss had left and I had been thrown into the editing chair until a replacement could be found. It was a fabulous distraction. The job was demanding and enjoyable, and I could forget about myself for hours on end. When I was ill, I had been inundated with advice about cutting back on my hours, going part-time, but, in fact, the opposite, working harder, proved the better antidote to depression for me.

In the June, it briefly looked as though my new temporary job would come to an end. I was summoned to see David English who, as far as I was concerned, ran the company. English was a smoothie, with that sleek, shiny look that successful men often have. Rupert Murdoch has it. From a distance, they look boring, another man in another suit, but close up you start to notice that they are not like other men at all. Their hair is always exactly the right length, their nails are short, but not too short, and startlingly clean, their pores are clean, their dull suits fit perfectly and their shirts have that just-out-of-the-packet-sheen. There's a slight, but only slight, hint of a tan. The man with a serious tan is a different, dodgier prospect altogether.

English was also consistently genial, polite in an almost self-conscious, mannered way that bordered on the ironic. But he was a powerful figure and many people were afraid of him. I wasn't, but his detached manner unsettled me, sometimes made me feel like a lower, messier form of life which, sadly, had to be tolerated for the sake of the newspaper. I never felt I quite came up to scratch with my bad-hair days and substandard pores. Whereas he was the archetypal hands-free executive, I always seemed to be loaded down with a giant handbag masquerading as a briefcase, a carrier bag with a few hasty purchases for home banging against my calf and a barely controlled bundle of papers and magazines wedged in my armpit. His office was at the top of the building and I often felt I was doomed to a life on the lower floors.

His assistant, more Miss Moneypenny than Bubble, was fabulously, almost defiantly, old school with her bouffant hair and vivid make-up. She always made me feel welcome. She occupied a large office – larger than most on the editorial floors and about three times the size of mine. English's own office was hilariously large, fit for a tycoon. I'm sure it had a view, but I have no memory of it. If you are stuck in a cage with a puma, you tend to keep your eyes on the puma. What was memorable about the office though was its utter lack of personality. It was decorated in that standard upscale, quasi-antique office style – there was probably a wood-effect fridge somewhere – but there was no paperwork or clutter. It felt empty, echoey. It was hard to imagine anyone working in it. But perhaps all his work – his scheming, strategic planning, whatever you prefer to call it – went on in his head and his surroundings were meaningless. Many newspaper journalists are like that – unlike magazine journalists, who are frequently more interested in appearances than their work. They are indifferent to their surroundings. All they need is a computer and a phone and, as they usually work in huge open-plan offices, they learn to block out the world and concentrate. I have always been like that. I can work at home in the sitting room, with children's TV blaring in the background. It's not ideal and sometimes I fantasise about how wonderful it would be to have that perfect room of my own, but it doesn't bother me that much. The trouble is that most newspaper journalists and writers like me don't have assistants running round after us, so our offices – or perhaps that should be areas – tend to look like health hazards.

That day, when I was called into English's office, we sat at a low table. There was a tray with a teapot, cups and saucers, and some posh biscuits. I knew the form. When prompted, I would pour myself a cup of tea but would never get to drink it. I would be turfed out again before it was cool enough to drink. And the biscuits? Oh no. They were a ploy in the power game. Just as I was halfway through that extra-crumbly digestive, English would suddenly decide that it was my turn to speak and would wait oh-so-patiently, staring quizzically all the while, as I gulped and swallowed and took a few ineffectual swipes at the crumbs on my face and suit before blurting out my reply, a feeble version of my carefully prepared speech. So although I could have wolfed down the whole plate, I said, thank you, but no.

English rather formally asked after my health, my brush with death, as he called it, and we discussed John Diamond, the journalist who, at the time, was writing about his own experience of cancer in the *Times*. He said he disagreed with John who, apparently, had said that he didn't like the notion of a battle with cancer. English said that he thought it was a battle, a fight, and then asked me what I had learned from my brush with death. I waffled incoherently about the importance of family. I had, of course, learned quite a few things, but they were too vague and abstract, perhaps too poncy, for this kind of headlined conversation and to say that I had learned nothing would have seemed rude. Before I was dismissed, we briefly discussed the magazine and he said he would be putting his mind to its future. I never saw him again. The next day I learned that he had died.

It was an odd feeling. I was the one who was supposedly cosying up to death and there he was, dead. It seemed to have little to do with fighting and battles. At his memorial service, I was seated upstairs in a corner, way down the pecking order, so I didn't see the protester downstairs, hustled out after complaining about the treatment of gays in the company's newspapers, a battle of a different kind.

By then there was a new regime in place. The paper itself had a new editor, Peter Wright, and Paul Dacre – often referred to as Paulie on the magazine, after the gang leader in the film *Goodfellas* – had taken over English's uber-editorial role. In the January, I got a new boss and settled back into my deputy editor role. Throughout this upheaval, I had been approached by another newspaper and a magazine about work, but I wasn't looking to leave. My paper and my boss, Simon, had behaved impeccably, helpfully and with great patience towards me while I was ill. They were not warm and cuddly – they didn't call me or visit. But I was put under no pressure to return to work before I was ready and when I did return, I was allowed to gradually build up my hours. The managing director was also very supportive during my temporary editorship, as was Peter when he arrived. I appreciated these kindnesses enormously.

But in the summer of 2000, I was sitting in my office and took a call which, not immediately but eventually, was to change my working life. When I say office, I use the term loosely. The room was roughly four by seven and contained a desk, a typing chair, two shelves and a nasty bright blue armchair which looked like it had been chopped off a banquette in the waiting room of a cut-price solicitor. The partition wall behind my desk sliced across a window, affording me a partial but pleasant view of St Mary Abbots church on the corner of Kensington Church Street. If I swivelled round on my chair, I could rest my feet quite comfortably on the other three walls, something I did frequently, particularly when I was on the phone.

The caller was Paula Reed, whom I had met at the *Sunday Times*. She had been the paper's fashion director and I had been both the managing editor of the section of the paper she worked for and the editor of the magazine. She was now working at another magazine, but was also in the process of setting up the British branch of an American charity called Gilda's Club. Gilda's was well-established across America as a non-profit cancer support organisation with its headquarters in New York. It was named after the comedian Gilda Radner. I had been aware of the project, but only dimly. Halfway through my treatment, I had gone along with Lucian to a fundraising performance of *The Nutcracker* at the Coliseum and I had arranged for the magazine to run an interview with the charity's British patron, Pierce Brosnan, but neither contribution was exactly selfless and I was too preoccupied with myself to do much else. Paula filled me in.

Gilda had been a mainstay of the satirical TV show *Saturday Night Live* and was married to the actor Gene Wilder. When she was diagnosed with advanced ovarian cancer, she went to the pioneering Wellness Community in California which ran support groups for people with cancer. She also spent a lot of time on the east coast and was upset that she couldn't find the same level of support there, so when she died in 1989, Gene Wilder asked Gilda's cancer therapist, Joanna Bull, if she would be interested in moving to New York to remedy this. She was, and the idea they came up with was Gilda's Club, which opened in 1995 in Greenwich Village on West Houston Street. Since then clubs had sprung up all over America and Canada, offering support groups, lectures, workshops and social events for people with cancer, their families and friends, in welcoming, comfortable clubhouses, free of charge and, crucially, whatever the outcome. There was no suggestion that membership equalled survival. The aim was simply to provide a structure whereby people could build their own social and emotional support, and share their collective wisdom. It was, in many ways, a community centre, a cancer community centre.

Paula had met Joanna and visited the New York clubhouse when it was still a building site. She had read about Gilda's in one of the American papers not long after her sister Margot had died of Hodgkin's disease at just 29. She was so inspired by Joanna's vision and so convinced that she and her family would have benefited from the Gilda's support programme during Margot's illness that she decided to start raising money to establish a club in London. She used her contacts in the fashion world to attract support for the idea and, by the time I spoke to her, had established a small office with one member of staff. I listened carefully, but a little unsure as to why Paula was telling me all this. She then took me completely by surprise. She asked me if I would be interested in talking to her about running Gilda's Club in London.

Me? Work for a charity? I loved journalism and, in the main, journalists who, despite their terrible reputation, are generally sharp, funny and interesting. Sometimes the work is hard, really hard, but it's often exhilarating, rarely boring. There's always a new story to pump up the volume. I'd never been tempted to change career. I had also never felt the urge to 'give back' after having cancer. I was not brimming over with gratitude for the help I had been given or so angry about the help I had wanted but which was not available that I wanted to do something to ensure that everyone else got that help. I had, in no way, become more altruistic. There seemed to be an idea abroad that, whatever a person is like before they have cancer, afterwards they are transformed into some kind of saint. I am still waiting for this to happen or see it happen to anyone else, despite what I later did. The drive to 'give back' is not, I think, quite what it seems.

When I was growing up, giving was a given; not giving back, just giving. My mother believed in it passionately. I also went to an evangelical Sunday school – for no reason except that it was nearby and the pastor lived next door to us – and was roped into delivering Christian Aid envelopes. One week, we would schlepp the streets pushing them through letterboxes, the next we would collect them, heavy with three-penny bits and sixpences. At Christmas, my mother would produce one of these envelopes after lunch – it was one of the few times of the year when we children had any serious cash – and we would be asked if we had any presents that we didn't want as these could be given to charity, too. The message was clear: we were better off than many others and should do our bit. Another message – that there were many, many others who were better off than us – was completely beside the point. The only point worth discussing was that we had enough to give to others.

Enough. It is a concept I now struggle with. I am a child of the Sixties and my parents brought up five children on one modest salary. My father started out as a mechanical engineer, then became a college lecturer after training as a teacher as a mature student, while my mother ran the house. But when I was 11, we moved into a spacious house with a large garden. Four of us children went to university. When I read accounts of the Sixties, they resonate with my life as much as Margaret Mead's account of growing up in Samoa. Nobody I knew had a scrubbed pine kitchen table or went on the Aldermaston Marches. What I took from that decade was the idea that life was good and would simply carry on getting better and better. And so, of course, we had enough to help the starving African babies – probably from Biafra – blazoned all over those little envelopes.

It was 1975 when I went to university. My fees were paid, as were everybody's in those days; I was awarded nearly a full grant for my living expenses and my parents made a small contribution. I felt rich. I had no interest in stuff, but that wasn't so unusual back then. Some people had expensive record players, but there weren't many gadgets around and I never knew anyone who went shopping as a pastime, which is hard to imagine nowadays. As a teenager, I'd made some of my own clothes, which is also hard to imagine today, and I developed a passion for secondhand clothes, now laughably called vintage, which I could fix up. My money went on books, occasionally records and my social life. I was, in fact, quite poor, but it didn't feel like that.

The day after my finals finished I started work and I've not stopped since. I have a strong work ethic. As a teenager, I found myself a Saturday job as soon as it was legal. I found Christmas and summer jobs throughout school and university. I thought it was perfectly normal that I had a job to go to as soon as finals were over. I was 20 and the only breaks I have had since then are my two brief maternity leaves, the eight months it took to have my cancer treatment and a six-month break in 2001. In some ways though, I think of my working life as starting when I joined the *Sunday Times* when I was 30. It was my first taste of hard work, 50- and 60-hour weeks and being shouted at all the time. It was also my first experience of a large and ever-growing salary. I spent nine years there, followed by four years at the *Mail on Sunday* where I earned even more money. And yet, after the initial thrill of having no money worries, these were the years when I never felt I earned enough. I always wanted more. I found it hard to resist the greedy, individualistic mantras of the time. I lost interest in giving money to charity. One Christmas I felt momentarily guilty and asked everyone to make a donation to Amnesty International instead of buying me a present and I once gave £300 to my university's alumni fund. Otherwise I probably gave about £100 a year to various charities, a pitiful percentage of my salary.

So when Paula asked me if I would be interested in working for Gilda's Club, I was taken aback. And, compared to what I was earning, the salary was laughable. Paula explained that she needed someone with management experience which I had in spades, someone who was good at team-building – she had seen me do this many times – and someone who knew about publicity and communications. She was not looking for someone who understood the nitty-gritty of fundraising. Someone else would be responsible for that. That answered my questions about why me. But I could not see myself becoming involved in the charity world, let alone the cancer world. I was still fixated on getting back to some kind of normal life and I felt convinced that my sanity depended on moving away from the cancer world, not becoming part of it. So it was pretty easy for me to say no to Paula, the first time at least.

The second time she asked was the following spring. By then I had left the newspaper and was working for a small start-up company on the launch of a new magazine. I had never worked for a small company before – all my jobs had been with big corporations. I had never had any illusions that small was beautiful, but this brief glimpse of life outside of the mainstream somehow made me more open-minded to Paula's project than I had been before. I was also, I felt, more detached from my own traumatic cancer experience. I wasn't actually, but I wasn't as depressed as I had been.

I was interviewed by one of the charity's trustees and made a formal offer. I was still nervous though, nervous about changing direction, the drop in salary and that working in the cancer world would reawaken some of my old anxieties. So when Paula suggested that she send me to Chicago to one of the Gilda's Club conferences so that I could meet the founder, Joanna Bull, and see for myself what the organisation was about, I leapt at the chance. I went with Sophie, that sole member of staff. Before Gilda's, Sophie had had a successful career in PR and, on the plane to Chicago, she told me about her mother's death from cancer and the effect it had had on her. She also filled me in on her Gilda's training in New York which I would have to undergo if I accepted the job. I was intrigued, my worries fading fast, and, within 20 minutes of arriving at the conference and meeting just a few of the Gilda's staff, I knew that I wanted the job. I wanted to be part of the Gilda's community. I could come up with a dozen reasons why I shouldn't get involved – the salary being top of the list – but I liked what I saw and heard, and I think there was an element of recklessness in my decision. Before I had been ill, I would have considered the long-term implications more seriously. Now that I was unable to think long-term, I simply thought, why not? I was, I knew, making a big change in my life, but despite what other people thought, it had nothing to do with giving back, seeing the light. If someone had offered me a job running an aquarium at this point, I may well have taken it. I was, of course, offered the Gilda's job partly because of my cancer experience and it's partly why I took it. But not entirely.

The deciding factor was meeting Joanna Bull, the founder of Gilda's Club. Joanna is one of those inspirational women. She's pretty, blonde, elegant and self-contained, and quite compelling. Later I discovered that she is a Buddhist, which partly explains her demeanour and attitudes. She has now retired from Gilda's, but at the time she was its figurehead and her sidekick was Joan Licursi, her opposite in so many ways, dark, flamboyant, funny and loud, to me the typical high-energy New Yawker. They were perfectly matched.

They asked Sophie and me to breakfast, one of those ludicrous pancake numbers so popular with American hotels. The waiter served me first and I thought he was giving me the whole order and that, for some unexplained reason, I had been chosen to be mother. I hadn't. It was just an obesity-special. I told Joanna that I was seriously interested in the job. She told me that she would be honoured if I would take it. It sounds cheesy. It's the kind of thing only an American could say without an ironic smile, but it was nice, a nice change from British cynicism. I returned home and handed in my notice at the magazine, and booked myself in for the Gilda's training programme in June in New York.

Despite being sure of my decision, I set off for New York – with the newly appointed programme director, Ray, a former cancer nurse and researcher – with a lorry-load of concerns, one of which was whether I could, at 42, share an apartment for two weeks with a man I hardly knew.

I wouldn't have missed it for anything. There were about 12 of us on the course; staff from clubs about to open and new staff from existing clubs. From nine to nine every day, we learned about the history, philosophy and programme structure of Gilda's. I learned to meditate, I learned to salsa (well, tried to), I went to a lymphoma networking group where I struggled with everyone else to understand blood tests, and I watched children having a ball in Noogieland, the play area where children go when their carers are using the club. Ray and I would get back to our rented apartment at about 9.30 and would slump into the comfortable armchairs, mulling over what we had learned as we demolished plates of pasta cooked in the primitive kitchen, washed down with Californian Merlot. Sometimes we even had pudding – Hershey bars. I think we got through Dean & Deluca's whole range of pasta sauces while we were there. It was student-life, the posh version.

The most moving part of the training for me was watching the support groups. These take many forms at Gilda's. There are groups for people with cancer; for people with a family member or friend with cancer; alumni groups for existing members who have either moved on from their initial diagnosis or lost someone to cancer; and for children. All are open to men and women, for people with all types of cancer. They are not therapy groups, simply a place where members share their thoughts.

I watched the adult groups through a two-way mirror, and sat in on a children's Small Talk group. I was astounded by the universality of the cancer experience. Regardless of age or diagnosis, members expressed remarkably similar fears, anger and feelings of isolation. They also, when we talked to them afterwards, said that when they had first come to Gilda's they were anxious, didn't know what to expect, but felt that it had changed their lives for the better. There was the relief, at first, of meeting people who knew exactly what they were going through and then, later, the enriching sense of friendship and community, the pleasure of sharing what they had learned with new members, which, in turn, made them realise how far they had come themselves. One member told me that he had changed his mind about leaving New York because there was no Gilda's Club where he had planned on moving.

Gilda's groups, however, are not warm and fuzzy hugathons of sharing – which I would have found repellent. As the programme director of New York, Harriet, told me in Chicago, death is the elephant in the room. Members often need to talk about it but, like most of us, don't know where to start. Some of the discussions were harrowing and there were a couple of times in New York when I thought I would lose it. In one group, I watched a woman my age who had just been treated for cervical cancer talk about how her prognosis was poor and that she had a small child. I have got to survive, she said. She was off the Richter scale with anxiety. But I saw her transformed by listening to a volunteer talk about her own experience. As I left the club that evening, I saw her smiling. At no point did anyone suggest that long-term survival was possible for everyone, but the meeting had given this woman the sense that someone else had been where she was now and that there could be hope. And hope, as I knew, however fragile and compromised it may be, is what we all need to get up in the morning.

Observing the Small Talk group was one of the hardest things I have ever done. It was thought inappropriate for us trainees to watch the group through the two-way mirror, so a couple of us sat in on the group. I was frightened that I would cry and upset the children. There were four in the group and they sat round a table with Laura, the facilitator. I met two girls of around my children's ages whose mother had recently died. They had come to the club with their father and been asked to bring something that reminded them of her. They had brought a photo album. I was humbled by their dignity, and the sensitivity and lack of probing by Laura. A little boy, whose father had died, brought in his father's hat which he liked to wear because the smell reminded him of his dad. Afterwards, they ran off laughing to Noogieland, looking as though they didn't have a care in the world. It doesn't get any better than this, I thought.

Joanna's belief is that social and emotional support enables people to live with cancer, rather than existing with it, and that the clubhouse is where they can structure that support. This structure is important and seeing how it worked brought home to me how I had struggled with this issue. I had received excellent medical care, but I had felt, so often, emotionally stranded. Throughout my treatment, I had wanted to talk to people going through the same thing, as did Simon, but how? I tried befriending patients in the clinic, but it wasn't easy with everyone wound up about their appointment. I was eventually plugged into a network of friends, and friends of friends, and eventually I found a therapist. But it was a painfully slow process. Simon's needs always got shoved into second place which was tough. Gilda's would have handed us both support on a plate.

It would also have helped everyone else in my circle. Joanna firmly believes that when cancer happens, it happens to the whole family, not just blood family but all those who are close to us. I had been protected from much of their anxiety when I was ill, but some of the fallout couldn't be hidden from me. Once my treatment was over and I started to recover, I gradually became aware of the physical and emotional exhaustion of those who had supported me. Simon became withdrawn for a while, shell-shocked. My mother took to her bed when she got a cold, something she never normally did. I heard whispers of my sisters – and many friends – trying to persuade hospitals to give them mammograms despite the fact that they were under 50. My sister Sarah, who had been depressed, became more so briefly. My sister Nellie told me later that she nearly walked out of a film because she suddenly realised that one of the characters had breast cancer. And these were the things I heard about. I can only imagine the more profound effects my illness had on them and which they were loath to burden me with. Watching the support group for family and friends during my training, I listened to the anxieties, the anger, the fears. It was difficult. I felt, all over again, so guilty and saw how much support everyone needed, not just me.

Everyone on the course was affected by the support groups, but many of them had counselling or, like Ray, medical experience. Their professional backgrounds had taught them about boundaries. I was, I felt, affected by them in a different way. I didn't seem to have any boundaries. And this worried me. I was being asked to do a job, not to sit around empathising. Joanna had a rule of thumb that people should not work at Gilda's, even in a voluntary capacity, unless they were a year on from their diagnosis or experience of cancer. I think I had followed this rule instinctively and cautiously when I had turned down Paula's first offer. But, three years on, I still did not feel in the clear. I was worried that I would feel overwhelmed by people's problems. I also worried that I was attracted to the job because I was looking for support for myself.

In the end, it was fine. It was Ray's job to deal with the members directly. It was mine to make sure that everything was in place so that Ray could do that job efficiently and appropriately. I talked to members if I bumped into them in the clubhouse or when I attended the odd workshop or lecture, but I did not seek them out. Each week, Ray and I met to discuss the membership but our discussions were about practical issues, making sure we had the right facilitators for the groups, that we were running the right kind of groups, about publicising the groups. And was I supported? Of course I was, but indirectly, in that Gilda's normalised and demystified the cancer experience for me. It also reinforced a growing belief that cancer is a common experience made difficult by the myths and taboos we have about it in our society.

I had, by the time I took the job, been in therapy for three years and I knew it was helping me. Gilda's showed me how it could, in a slightly different form, help others. People were often tentative coming through the door. It's not easy to admit that, yes, you really do have cancer and, yes, you do need support. Once they crossed the threshold though, it was difficult to get them to leave. The relief at being able to talk openly about their cancer, their fears, was tangible. It also seemed to give them permission to laugh – like me, when their lows were silenced, so were the highs.

171

Gilda's reinforced my belief that support should be of a high standard, regulated. The facilitators were carefully vetted and given supervision – a convention whereby therapists see a therapist themselves. Ray, because of the front-line nature of his work, also qualified for supervision. I felt comfortable with this system and was often alarmed when I met representatives of other support organisations who were laid back, even ignorant about the most basic guidelines on support work. It is still the case in this country that I could call myself a counsellor, never having done a day's training. Other counsellors are trained but their qualifications may not be recognised by the bodies governing therapeutic practice. Some self-help groups round the country run telephone counselling and support groups without any knowledge of this practice. Are they better than nothing? I'm not sure. Some people are, by nature, empathic, non-judgemental, supportive. Others are just busy-bodies with weird hang-ups and opinions about cancer that are misguided. They love a crisis and can be more dangerous than helpful.

The standards and structure of Gilda's were developed to avoid this kind of madness. The groups of around 10 people are run by a therapist called a facilitator who is there to anchor the group. They do not offer up any topics of conversation or interpret what is said. They simply announce when they think everyone is ready to start and, two hours later, draw the meeting to a close. The members talk to each other, not the facilitator, and it is up to them to decide what they speak about and how. The only times during my training that I ever saw a facilitator intervene were to ask someone who had not spoken if they wanted to say something, to suggest that everyone not talk at once and, once, to ask the group why they were being so critical of the wife of one of the group's members who was dying in hospital. The facilitator makes the group feel safe, but the facilitator's back seat approach also makes it feel in control, a rare feeling when you are dealing with cancer.

A lot of doctor-bashing goes on, some of which is justified and some of which is simply a channel for inchoate anger. Doctors are not paranoid when they say that's what support groups get up to. But from what I saw in America and what I heard from Ray about the London groups, more doctor-bashing goes on in America. I have some rich friends and if they ever talk about cancer, they say that if they are ever diagnosed they will jump on a plane to New York and go to Sloan-Kettering, the cancer hospital there. Apart from the cost – I don't think even rich people realise just how expensive cancer treatment is – the way the American medical system works is daunting to say the least.

My cancer treatment was carried out in three hospitals – Charing Cross, Hammersmith and the Cromwell – but it was overseen by the same medical team, experienced doctors who had opinions about what the best treatment was for me. Once I had been referred by my GP, I was in their hands and they all knew what was happening to me at any given time. In America, patients pretty much supervise their own care, finding their own surgeons, oncologists, radiotherapists, etc., all of whom may be in different places. They lug round great files of notes and X-rays and test results, and worry constantly about whether their insurance will cover this or that particular doctor, treatment or test. They also, of course, take responsibility for deciding themselves which doctors, treatments or tests are appropriate. It is a huge responsibility.

The people I met at Gilda's in New York thought our health service was rubbish, couldn't imagine not having choice, but, to me, their choice came with a heavy price. If your health insurance was not the best, your choice was limited. I heard terrible stories of impersonal, production-line care and people being sent home immediately after operations because they couldn't afford to stay in overnight. The latter brought back memories of a terrifying account I had read many years before by the writer Kathy Acker who had a double mastectomy as day surgery for this reason. And even if your health insurance is good, you still have to devote enormous resources to organising your medical care and you have to know what you are looking for, what you want. Our health service is far from perfect, not everyone is treated in big London teaching hospitals as I mainly was, and not everyone is able to be as pushy as you often need to be to get what you need, but I'm not sure how most of us would fare in the jungle of the American system. So I wasn't surprised to see support groups discussing their care – or lack of it – at such length.

Both in New York and London though, members talked mainly about their fears and about death. Sometimes that is sad, but more often it is liberating. It's what you think about when you or a loved one has cancer, and pretending you aren't is exhausting. I knew this from my own experience but I was also moved seeing how it worked for others, how voicing fears lessened them. I could see it in people's posture. They became less hunched, less defensive. I could hear it in their voices which became louder, stronger.

The real tragedy is that there is so little opportunity for people to get this kind of support. When you are diagnosed with cancer, if you are lucky, you are offered a number of services at the hospital. At Charing Cross, I had access to a relaxation class, a set number of massage or reflexology sessions and counselling. This service is exceptional and I took advantage of it. At the Cromwell, I was again offered counselling which I took up. Once my treatment was finished, however, I was on my own. I did continue seeing the counsellor, Sally Parr, at the Cromwell but I then had to pay for the sessions. I know why this happens. Funding isn't endless. But the problem is that, although help is wonderful when you are going through treatment, it is, in some ways, more useful afterwards when you are no longer under the supervision of the doctors, and feeling at your most vulnerable and alone with your cancer. Gilda's, I felt, could step in and fill this gap in the cancer support network.

There is also something about the social aspect of Gilda's that is unusual. The kitchen is always open with tea, coffee and water. There are different places to sit – sofas and tables and chairs. In New York, I met three women who took their lunch to the club each week before their support group. It was a place where people can truly be themselves. Everybody knows why they are there, so a whole level of social awkwardness falls away, and with it, the social isolation that comes with cancer. They don't have to keep up any kind of front. I saw the same thing happen in London. Nobody gawped at anyone who was bald or too thin. Everyone understood fatigue, dodgy stomachs. (Clubhouses have lavatories with proper walls – when you are ill, there's nothing more embarrassing than a flimsy partition wall round a lavatory.) In London, people popped in before or after hospital appointments. They found it welcoming, relaxing. They would make themselves a cup of tea, sit on the sofa by the large fish tank, chatting, reading magazines. I never experienced a moment of doubt about the services Gilda's offered. Intellectually, they were well thought out. Practically, they were a hit with members. But not all my experiences there were good. I was often shocked by the charity world itself.

My first shock was the people. Having spent my adult working life in magazines and newspapers, with pushy, sharp, egotistical types, I was now faced with a different type of person altogether, quieter, slower. I was used to a rough-and-tumble work environment where people shouted a lot, were outrageously un-PC and generally difficult. Now I found myself in an environment where political correctness was a given and people liked rules and regulations, detailed job descriptions, mountains of paperwork. I spent so much time writing letters. Phone calls and emails were, apparently, not the thing. I liked the people I worked with, particularly Ray and, later, Karen who came to help with fundraising. My friend Anna also, through a strange sequence of events, became the clubhouse manager. But I often found the world we operated in dour, hidebound, rigid and slow. I had to adapt fast and my sister Nellie, who had always worked in the public sector, found my frustrations amusing, particularly the earnestness. Once Ray and I went to a conference together and, as we sat down in the lecture theatre, I turned to him and said, 'For the first time in my life I feel like a supermodel.' It was a ridiculous thing to say but it's how I felt. Everyone looked so ferociously sensible.

These people, I knew, were the backbone of the charity world. They were the ones who slogged away, badly paid, for the good of others. I was a newcomer, a know-nothing. What had I ever done for anyone? Eighteen months later when I left Gilda's I still felt frustrated by the earnestness of these people and I didn't warm to many of them, but I developed a great deal of respect for their doggedness, their ability to keep going. Horses for courses, perhaps. But I also realised that they were not quite what they seemed. At first, I presumed that their modesty reflected their altruism. Although I doubted my own motives for working for a charity, I had not doubted the motivation of anybody else. I thought, I suppose, that they were simply better, kinder people than me. I soon realised that their motivation was often as complicated as mine was.

There were those who fell into the 'giving back' category, who had had their own cancer experiences and now wanted to help others. Some of these people were calm and reasonable. Others were a mass of neuroses, unresolved guilt, anxiety and anger. Then there were those who had not had any cancer experience but had a non-specific desire to work for a charity, any charity. Again, some of these people were entirely reasonable. Others were damaged, finding relief in helping those they saw as even worse off than themselves. In other words, most of the people I met got something out of what they did. They were not saints, or at least I never met any.

Another group of people I had to deal with was equally challenging – the ladies who lunch and the celebrities who were supposed to help Gilda's raise money. Some were delightful, modest and hard-working, the kind of people who never wanted their name bandied about, just wanted to help with contacts and write cheques. Others were appalling, promising lots and then leaving Gilda's staff to do the real work, or gushing to the press about their amazing charity work when all they had done was attend a fundraising dinner. Some didn't even want to pay for these dinners, thinking that their presence was their contribution. I was told by those with more experience than me that this was not unusual and to shut up. But I was uncomfortable with it because I saw the generous donations from ordinary people, people with comparatively little money.

Large charities employ people whose job it is to deal with socialites and celebrities, and I take my hat off to them. It's a difficult job, but someone has to do it. With our cronky old class system and our obsession with celebrity, the rich and famous are seen as useful to charities for publicity. During my time at Gilda's I was rung daily by companies suggesting that they would raise money for us or make a donation if we would lend them one of our famous supporters or let them use our name to approach other celebrities who would endorse some product or other. Other companies wanted to organise launch parties and needed well-known faces to attract press photographers. Sometimes these weird arrangements worked. Gilda's got some money, the celebrities got their pictures in the paper. Sadly though, most of the calls I took were about the one A-list celebrity connected to Gilda's, Pierce Brosnan, who was, at that point, unavailable for appearances.

Gilda's HQ in New York found it strange, couldn't understand why these names didn't make personal donations to Gilda's. In America, the system is much more straightforward: you get involved with a charity and you give or get, i.e. get money from others. The fact that there are good tax breaks for charitable giving is an incentive, as is the fact that there is no national health service. In America, it is considered extra-ordinary that Gilda's is free. In London, it was simply taken for granted. There are more rich people in America than here, but there is also a different attitude. The various Gilda's Clubs round the country were franchises, self-funding, and were often kick-started by seed money from individual philanthropists. Other people then came on board and did more giving and getting. None of them wanted their name over the door. Many of them were Jewish. I met a handful at the various conferences I went to and was struck by their quiet generosity.

I was aware that I was only scratching the surface of the giving culture in America and that maybe there were more similarities than I could see, but what was indisputable was that the Americans I met were not embarrassed about money, at least not in the way that British people are. They didn't cringe at the thought of asking wealthy or famous people for money and those who were asked for money apparently didn't cringe either, seemed to expect to be asked. There are protocols for making the ask, as it's called, but it is not as loaded as it is here. Back in London, I felt we were in the dark ages, doffing our caps to toffs in the hope of a few small crumbs or, more often, pandering to the whims of the almost-famous for a photo-caption in the *Standard* which might – or might not – mention Gilda's Club. This 'might not' was always a risk because some supporters, when I met them, seemed to know very little about Gilda's, had no interest in knowing more and certainly no interest in seeing the club or meeting any of the workers. My natural indifference to the celebrity culture was slowly transformed into loathing. One of the last straws was being shouted at down the phone by a celebrity who had agreed to be interviewed about Gilda's and had earlier turned down my offer of being talked through the charity's brief history and aims. She now wanted to take me up on that offer, but insisted that it could not be done over the phone and that I had to go to her house early the very next morning. She did not ask nicely.

The people I ended up admiring, apart from the hard-working backroom workers, were the large charities such as Macmillan who help out smaller charities, the rich people who set up trusts – bodies to which charities apply formally for funding – and ordinary people who put their hands in their pockets, or go on fun runs, organise jumble sales and rattle tins. There are also the supermarkets, banks and big companies who give large amounts of money and make impressive efforts to publicise the charity to their staff and customers. Others help on projects which are hard to get funding for – one large bank helped Gilda's with photocopying, a mailout and printing a leaflet. It expected nothing in return.

Gilda's closed after 18 months in the autumn of 2001 because of a funding crisis. Money was simply not coming in fast enough. I was sad. Paula had worked so hard to set it up. All of us who worked at the club had thrown ourselves into the project. The services it offered were, I think, without parallel in cancer support. My feeling as I locked the door behind me for the last time was that it was a great loss to people with cancer, their families and friends. I altered my list of things I would do if I won the lottery to include setting it up again. But I also thought I could never work for a charity again. I would give money when I could, but I would, I thought, once I'd recovered, go back to journalism.

In fact, it took me six months to relaunch myself. I felt

bruised, confused, but I did go back to journalism. I'm glad. I feel I fit in better in that world. I became a different kind of journalist though. I became a freelance writer and editor, something I would never have considered before as it is so precarious, often appallingly paid. One of the reasons was that I had been told by some people I approached about work that their newspapers might be leery of giving a staff job to someone with my health record, something which is impossible to prove either way given the quixotic way in which most people are given jobs in journalism. But somehow, having made one big career change – and drop in salary – made it easier to contemplate another. It was yet another example of the impossibility of ever really going back for me. And, hardly surprisingly given my track record on resolutions, I soon found myself involved with the charity world again.

I had, when I was at Gilda's, filled in a form for CancerBACUP, the cancer information service, offering to read – from a patient's perspective – booklets for them. It seemed like something I could do which utilised both my cancer experience and my journalistic skills. But I had heard nothing from them and had forgotten about my offer. Then, last year, I suddenly started receiving regular packages from them. I would read a booklet – say, on Advanced Cancer or Breast Cancer – make my comments and send them back. I was then asked if I would join the Service Users' Forum, a group of patients who meet a couple of times a year to discuss various issues the charity is considering.

Around this time, Karen, the fundraiser whom I had worked with at Gilda's and who had become a friend, rang me out of the blue. I never would have met someone like Karen if I had not left journalism and that would have been my loss. She is one of those entirely reasonable people who like working for charities. She was helping a charity called the Cancer Counselling Trust and had discovered that they were looking for new trustees. Would I be interested? I wasn't sure. She asked if I would mind if she gave them my address so that they could send me some information. I didn't.

A few weeks later I received a large envelope with heaps of information about the charity. It offered, as its name suggests, one-to-one counselling for people with cancer or anyone touched by cancer. It also offered telephone and bereavement counselling. Fees were on a sliding scale with no one turned away for financial reasons. The counsellors were all trained and had once worked for CancerBACUP. When CancerBACUP decided that it could no longer offer counselling and wanted to concentrate on its information services, the counsellors formed CCT. It was now at a stage where it had its own premises, had an administrative structure, was offering a comprehensive counselling service and was starting to work with other organisations who needed advice and training in this kind of counselling work. It had also decided that it needed to appoint an executive director. It was growing slowly and sensibly. I could see why Karen had thought of me. It was a good fit.

Jane from the office rang me and we talked. I liked her. She had a good sense of humour. I went to a drinks party the charity held at its annual conference. I liked the people I met. I agreed to attend three trial trustees' meetings in order that both I and the other trustees could decide if the relationship could work. I felt completely at home with the charity's aims, but I was still anxious. Was I doing the right thing? Would this be Gilda's all over again? What did I have to offer? What was my motivation? Was I looking, vicariously, for support again? I wasn't worried about finding it depressing because my experience at Gilda's had shown me that this kind of work is challenging, inspiring and it isn't depressing. I was a little anxious about the worthy factor again, but at least there didn't seem to be any socialites or celebrities involved.

During my first two meetings, I realised that what I had to offer was simple: my experience at Gilda's – the successes, the failures – my enthusiasm and, lastly, my own cancer experience. I liked the staff, the other trustees. The more I learned about the service, the more I knew how important it was that it expand. Emotional support for anyone touched by cancer had improved a little since the demise of Gilda's, but not enough. CCT decided that the relationship would work and in October 2003 I became a trustee. I felt a deep sense of satisfaction that something valuable had come out of my experiences. It made me think about when I first met Julie Friedeberger at the Yoga Therapy Centre back in 2000. During relaxation she asked us to think of a word to meditate on. Completely unbidden, the word 'open' came into my mind and now it did again. You can make plans, I thought, but if you close yourself off from new experiences, are not open to them, you just might miss out on some of the best things in life.

I still feel sad that Gilda's didn't work out. Clients at CCT often say they would like somewhere to decompress after their counselling, to have a cup of coffee. A clubhouse is a good idea.

It also builds community. Few of us live in communities now, especially in cities. Most of the time, we feel this lack of community in vague ways, but illness makes us feel it sharply, and although a cancer community is a club we instinctively feel we don't want to join, if we can put aside our misgivings for long enough to give it a whirl, we may find ourselves pleasantly surprised. It's what seems to have happened to me. I've not so much given back as been given something. This doesn't mean that I am glad I had cancer – I am not – just that some of the side-effects, although they do not in any way negate the pure horror of the experience, have been quite wonderful.

8

The Passenger

While I have been writing this book, I have been haunted by the thought of one day getting up, sitting at my computer and writing the words: 'And then it came back.' My progress has also been frustratingly lacking in any linearity. I have not gradually increased in confidence. I've lurched and lolloped. My five-year check-up was a big downer.

I was sitting in Mr Sinnett's office, the same office where I was diagnosed. He was smiling. My scans were clear. I heard the phrases 'good news' and 'doing so well'. My response? I burst into tears. And I wasn't crying with relief, I was crying because I was frightened.

This was not supposed to happen. This was my five-year check-up. I had reached the big one, the one that gets mentioned in all the statistics, the one that everyone thinks is the holy grail, the thinking being that if you have had five years without a relapse, you are cured. I should have been pleased, thrilled even. I should have been dancing around like Woody Allen in *Hannah and Her Sisters* when he finds out that he does not, after all, have a brain tumour. Instead, I kept rewinding the tape to the bit where he walks despondently down the street, jostled by indifferent passers-by, convinced that he is going to die.

Mr Sinnett was sympathetic, but perplexed. He reiterated the good news stuff with all the provisos which are thrown into the pot when my doctors talk to me about my cancer. I listened carefully, but I knew the facts. I knew that, despite what the general public thinks, I was not home and dry because I had been cancer-free for five years. My cancer could still come back at any time. But I also knew that five years was a milestone. I had been told that two years is statistically significant, as is three years, then five years, and that the longer I had no symptoms, the less aggressive my cancer and the more successful my treatment is presumed to have been. In short, I was not dying as far as anyone could tell and I should be delighted. But somehow I had managed to persuade myself that five years was not good news, but bad news.

This check-up took place in spring 2002. Everything I had learned about having cancer up to that point suggested that the experience was unlike anything I had heard or read about, so logically, the five-year check-up was bound to be different from the champagne-popping event of popular myth, too. But I was surprised by my extreme reaction to it and quickly realised that however determined I was to walk into each new experience with my eyes wide open and leave the corny expectations at the door, I wasn't always going to manage it. Even after five years, surviving cancer was proving to be a skill, maybe even an art, which I was still learning. A couple of months before this check-up, I would have said I was ready to try a few black runs, maybe even go off-piste, but now I wasn't so sure. In fact, I started wondering whether I would ever graduate from the nursery slopes. I was still, in so many ways, hung up on the idea that, somehow, I could crack this cancer thing.

I tried putting this check-up into the context of other, less loaded check-ups. It didn't help. They had all been ghastly and had not become noticeably easier. The only thing that had really changed over the years was that I had fewer check-ups. I once saw a flyer on Professor Coombes' desk, which I read upside down as I did with many scribbles and notes on doctors' desks. It was for women who had reached the five-year point, informing them that they no longer needed to come for check-ups at all, but to report in if they had any symptoms. I asked if I would be given this leaflet. No, I was told. We prefer to keep seeing the high-dose patients unless you really would prefer not to be seen. Naturally, I did and I didn't. I wanted to feel that someone was looking out for me, but I still hated the process.

In the run-up to each appointment, I would become irritable, anxious. Simon would try valiantly to reassure me. 'If there is anything wrong with you, you would probably know,' he would say. 'The fact that you are due for a check-up is neither here nor there. It's just a formality.' I knew this, of course, but I never seemed to be able to believe it. I had, when I first knew about the check-up system, thought that my appointments would involve elaborate tests and scans, long consultations. They didn't. When I saw Professor Coombes, I had a blood test and breast examination. When I saw Mr Sinnett, I had a mammogram, ultrasound and breast examination. Both felt my neck, tapped my back and chest, and poked around my stomach area. They also asked me how I was, in much the same way that anyone you bump into in the street does. It's a question I found hard to answer. Usually, I opted for the rather non-committal response of, 'Okay, I think.' Apparently, people like me used to be scanned regularly but the practice was halted when it was discovered that not only did the scans cause enormous stress, but patients were also reporting symptoms before the scans showed anything. So now the check-ups are simpler and, it is hoped, less highly charged. These considerations mean little to me. I cannot imagine check-ups being more highly charged than they are.

Apart from the pre-appointment anxiety, the rush of adrenalin during the appointment, I always feel awful afterwards. Sometimes I burst into tears in the corridor. I was exhausted, I craved chocolate croissants, sleep. It is as if, each time, I was being led in front of that firing squad and given a reprieve, and it was only the doctors who could give me that reprieve. I have no trust in anybody else's judgement or in my own instincts. The sting is that although I hate the check-ups, I also crave the fleeting reassurance they give me. Once I recover from them, I feel briefly elated, energised. Alive, I suppose.

Although it is unsettling that there seems to be no learning curve with my check-ups, I do understand why I am still blindsided by them. Over the years, I have come to see my cancer diagnosis as a large stone lobbed into the still pond that was my life, although back then I would have had trouble recognising such a description of it. As this stone hit the pond, it displaced a great deal of water. Everyone rushed to see what was happening. Then, as the stone sank from view, everyone lost interest. I thought I would, too. What I hadn't taken into consideration was the ripple effect. Over the years, these ripples became almost imperceptible, but they were there if you looked carefully and they have gradually covered the whole pond. As time has passed, I have gone for longer and longer periods of not noticing the ripples. The check-ups though – whatever mood I am in – have forced me to confront them.

The five-year check-up, however, was the worst. I felt awful. A fog descended on my brain. I could not think straight. Walking along the street one day – I can remember the exact spot, in Wright's Lane, a hundred yards from High Street Kensington, by the side entrance to Boots, a place which now always unnerves me – I wasn't sure whether I could put one foot in front of the other, whether I could go on. The burden was too much. I had, I felt, tried so hard to move on, to live with my cancer, and had got nowhere. I also convinced myself that five years was pushing my luck. From the outset, expectations for me seemed modest. Every symptom-free check-up was seen as a gift, not a given. So, I reasoned, my luck had to run out sometime. Why not now?

Mr Sinnett understood this sort of mad-thinking. He asked me if I would prefer to have my annual check-ups at a different clinic so that there would not be so many reminders of our first meeting when I was diagnosed. I said I would think about it. What I actually went home and thought about, though, was whether I had learned to hope, but not too much. The conclusion I came to was that I had hopes, but not expectations. At least that is what the rational part of my mind concluded. Alongside that ran a different narrative, one in which I was bargaining for my life. It was a fantasy, of course. I'm not sure with whom I had been or was still trying to strike a bargain, but I was definitely negotiating with someone. I'm not sure either what I was offering in return for life. I just know that something was going on, something definitely irrational, possibly bonkers, but nevertheless powerful. My wish, when I was diagnosed, was simple and has remained unchanged: I wanted to live long enough to see my children grow up. As they were six and three when I was diagnosed, this was a tall order. It was also, I now realised, rather dodgy in its non-specificity. When are children considered grown-up? When I had my five-year check-up, Lucian was 11 and Cosima eight. Had the bargain been fulfilled, I wondered? Or would my time be up when Cosima was 11? When they were both at secondary school, at university? When they had left home? When they had found their one true love? Could I renegotiate? I didn't think so. That scythe seemed to hover over my bowed, depressed head.

Strangely, this feeling was laced with guilt at having survived. Why me? The feeling had reared its head before when meeting friends or colleagues whose friends, sisters had not survived breast cancer. I felt awkward, too lucky. How to comport myself? How not to come across as smug, despite feeling nothing of the sort? It reminded me of the time when Lucian was a baby and, searching for the baby clinic at the hospital, I burst in on the AIDS clinic instead. There I was, brandishing, it suddenly seemed, this bouncing, bonny boy in the faces of rows of emaciated men.

You may think that it's morbid to dwell on these issues. I think it's facing up to reality. Two of the three women who had had breast cancer and supported me when I was diagnosed, Jackie and Katy, are now dead. Both died young, their cancer coming back in different, dangerous places, and Katy left two small children. I still have the letter from her which she sent just as I was going into chemo. Back then, it felt like she was throwing me a lifejacket. She cheered me on, encouraging me to believe that there was life after breast cancer. And she was right. It's just that there wasn't so very much of it for her and it was, for me, confirmation that, yes, the worst can happen. I tried to glean something from the wreckage of her life. When she knew she was dying, she told me not to call any more, to enjoy my life, forget about her. I miserably respected her wishes.

Other kinds of death have affected me differently. When Liz Tilberis, the editor of American *Harper's Bazaar*, wrote her book about having ovarian cancer, she noted how strange it felt when her friends Princess Diana and Gianni Versace, the fashion designer, died unexpectedly. She was the one who was supposed to be dead. My first experience of this feeling was slightly less glamorous. I was on the way to see Mrs Witham one afternoon in a cab when I heard on the radio that the journalist Jill Dando had been shot outside her house in Fulham. I was, like most people, deeply shocked but my shock was tempered with an unattractive triumphalism. She's dead. I'm not. I had a different reaction when my brother-in-law David died at 49 and, six months later, my father at just 70. Then I simply felt as though I had been beaten up in a backstreet alleyway and left to crawl home through unfamiliar streets.

And yet I know that I now have an understanding of life and death which is not shared by most people, however much they protest otherwise. It's the difference between actually being a parent and thinking you know what it's like because your friends have children who you see occasionally. And, in the same way that parenthood forces you, often slowly and painfully, to see the world and your place in it differently, so does illness. It's up to me now to monitor my health sensibly, not to over-react, but not to ignore warning signs. Sometimes I do this well, sometimes, like before my five-year check-up, I falter. As I say, it's an art surviving cancer.

I have on my desk a postcard of a photograph which I saw at the Sam Taylor-Wood exhibition at the Hayward. *Self-portrait in a Single-breasted Suit with Hare*, it says on the back. I love it. I love the play on words and the look in her eyes, the way she stares into the camera. She went through cancer treatment. It's a beautiful photograph but it's also, to me, unflinching. Here is life and here is death, it seems to say. There's an honesty about it that I like, that I rarely encounter in the real world. Sometimes I'm complicit, though, I admit. Like when someone says, 'Hi, how are you?' 'Fine,' I say. Sometimes, I actually mean it. But sometimes, I'm lying. My pants are on fire, ablaze.

Mr Sinnett says the next stage for me is 10 years, not eight or nine years. I'll be 49 then, nearly 50. It sends shivers down my spine even to write those words. It seems like tempting fate. But if it does come to pass, maybe I will be a little more sanguine, more positive about the future. I am still plagued by the same worries I had at the beginning of this nightmare journey. When my treatment finished, I could not imagine a future for myself at all and I couldn't plan ahead. Over the years, I have learned to look further ahead than tomorrow, but only to a few months hence. A couple of years ago, I booked a holiday in Italy. The booking was made in the New Year. The holiday was in June. No big deal to most people. I would never have done it if my sister Nellie had not suggested it, organised most of it. It felt like sticking my head above the parapet. I've never bothered to organise a personal pension since I abandoned the corporate world. I can't convince myself that I'll ever need one. I'd like to move, but I am frightened of moving away from the doctors who saved my life, the cutting-edge London hospitals. I've heard all those stories about postcode lotteries.

I worry most though about being ill. I am terrified of it in a way that I wasn't first time round. I worry about who will look after me. My fantasy is that, somehow, I would have enough money to have a nurse, which is highly unlikely. I've seen what happens when partners become nurses. Some are good at it, most aren't. It causes horrible tensions, maybe not of Baby Jane proportions, but bad enough. I also feel I've used up my sympathy quota with my family, with Simon, so I worry that I would languish in bed, miserable, acutely aware of the strain my illness was putting on family life, guilt preventing me from asking for what I really need and want. The word languish is important because the other terror that haunts me is the intense boredom and frustration of illness, the dependence on others, which can be humiliating, the watching of the clock, the struggle to please everyone by staggering downstairs to sit on the sofa for a while and, worst of all, the feeling of being trapped, a prisoner in my own home, an overgrown adolescent.

There is the anxiety, too, that things would be worse than before because, in all likelihood, there would be even less hope second time round and there would certainly be less money. I was cushioned by a company's generous sick-pay scheme before. This time I'd be on my own.

And what would I be thinking, if I could think straight? I would, I am sure, be trying to look on the bright side, to look at how much the last seven years have meant to me, how lucky I was to have had those years. I would also be thinking that I was lucky to have had the time to make sense of my life in therapy, a luxury denied those who die soon after their diagnosis. I would be thinking that old age had never looked much cop to me, that it was just a longer version of what I'd been through before and therefore I should be glad to forgo that experience. I would be thinking that I was glad that I had made the changes to my working life that I had, that having cancer had somehow given me the confidence to downshift, something I would otherwise have been even more nervous about than I was. Having cancer also, of course, made me unemployable in some people's eyes so the decisions I made were made in that context, but, being pragmatic, I had turned this disadvantage to my advantage, saw it as a chance to try new things.

And I am glad. When I was at the *Sunday Times*, one of my senior colleagues liked to make me, as he described it, wake up and smell the coffee. When I went back to work after Lucian was born, his only comment was, 'Just wait until he's 18 and asking you to drive him back to university and you have to tell him you can't because it's press night.' The thought of being in that or any similar office for another 18 years and the assumption that my son and everything else would always come second to my work horrified me, but I may well have stayed on. Plenty do. My colleague did, frequently lobbing me advice about topping up my pension. Sadly, he died before he got to use his.

My income is now comparatively low and my security has all but disappeared, but I have given myself a better quality of life. I spend more time with Simon and the children because I can fit my work round them now rather than vice versa. I have more time for reading, and meeting and phoning friends, and I have more friends, having more time to make and keep up friendships. I try to spend as much of my time as possible doing things that I think are important. These are simple things, but difficult to achieve when you are incarcerated in an office 50 hours a week. They're sometimes difficult to achieve even now. My life is a compromise, a bloody great compromise. A friend once told me that if she was ever diagnosed with cancer, she'd immediately take off on a hedonistic round-the-world trip. She didn't seem at all concerned about who would be looking after her daughter or paying the mortgage while she was jetting around, let alone about how ill she would probably be. She didn't understand that cancer doesn't stop all the clocks, but enough of them.

My approach seems to have been a watered-down version of *carpe diem*, seizing some of the day, perhaps just a few hours a day. It's a bit corny. If I had more money, I'd probably do less work, but I'd still do some because I believe that work is important to sanity. I'd probably take a course in philosophy, take a few holidays abroad and, instead of going to charity shops, I'd splash out on some Prada, the only designer who seems to understand women who don't want to look like tarts. But otherwise I'd do much the same as I do now. In fact, I'm more corny in other ways, too. When I became an aunt for the first time, to my sister Julie's daughter, Martha, I was delighted, to have a niece and to see my sister so happy. I also felt ridiculously lucky, footballer over-the-moon. I might never have lived to experience this, I thought. When it happened a second time, when my sister Sarah had her daughter Cicely, I felt doubly lucky.

When Kerry got married and invited me and Simon to be her and Jeremy's, well, everything at their quiet wedding, I was deeply moved. I felt proud of her looking so beautiful and happy, and felt the same all over again when she gave birth to her daughter Alicia. I also felt grateful to have lasted long enough to see her hit her stride so successfully.

It often takes a shock to shake us up in middle-age, not necessarily to make us realise What Really Matters – most of us know that already – but to stop for a while, reassess, make a few changes. The trouble is I could come up with a long list of shocks I would have preferred to a cancer diagnosis. Cancer is too loaded an issue, too weighted with symbolism, too scary, complicates things too much. A near-miss car crash would have been preferable perhaps. Or how about a breast lump that turned out to be benign? Because, to be frank, I am still furious that I was diagnosed with cancer. Whatever benefits there may have been, however lucky I sometimes feel I have been, these feelings are always outweighed by the distress my cancer has caused me over my beloved children.

9

Let's Stay Together

It was about halfway through my stem cell transplant when I reached rock bottom over Lucian and Cosima. I was feeling low. I had just opened a card from my friend Anna. Try to think about nice things, she said. Think about those times on the back steps in France. These words had transported me back to my twenties, to the many times when Anna and I had driven down to her parents' house in the Dordogne. There were no children then. We pleased ourselves, got up late, drinking coffee in the sun before drifting off to the local market, returning for a late lunch, a nap and hours of reading, Anna in the sun, me in the shade. Every evening, after a shower, we sat on the back steps where the sun lingered before it disappeared behind the vineyards, drinking chilled sweet Monbazillac, nibbling olives, talking about the books we were reading and snapping beans for supper which we would eat, well, whenever it was ready. These memories had made my hospital room seem even more claustrophobic, the view out of the window of grey sky and pylon even bleaker. I was overcome with despair. My situation felt untenable. I fought back tears of self-pity.

My mother was sitting by my side, reading the paper. She sensed my mood. I found it difficult to speak.

'This is so awful,' I said.

She took my hand.

'But,' I said, rallying suddenly, 'I think it would be worse if it was happening to one of the children. I don't know if I could bear that.'

'I know,' she said. 'I would do anything to swap places with you.'

I was taken aback by her answer. I had been so absorbed by my own feelings, my own misery, that I had not realised what I had said. I was mortified. I had been trying to convince myself that there were worse things than the situation I was in, to haul myself up from the bottom rung of the ladder of misfortune, but in doing so I had brought myself slap-bang up against one of my greatest fears, the fear that every mother has, the fear that I could not protect my children. When I was diagnosed, I immediately felt that I had ruined their lives, but I had not been able to examine that feeling. Every time I tried to, I ended up sobbing and my brain simply cut out. I had gone round and round in circles, trying to work out how to proceed as a mother, coming to no conclusions. The conversation with my mother – who else could it have been with, I now think – took me a step forward in my understanding.

We live in such a misogynistic society that it is often difficult to make sense of the mother–child relationship. There is no longer any consensus about what constitutes the good-enough mother. The old rules have been broken, replaced by claptrap. Whether we work or stay at home, there's always someone somewhere who is happy to tell us where we are going wrong – we work too much, too little, we worry about our children too much, too little. Embattled and confused, we muddle along, doing our best, making up our own rules, defining motherhood for ourselves. But when our backs are against the wall, the conflicting opinions and emotions, the frustrations become as nothing. For most of us, the relationship comes down to one thing: we will do anything to protect our children, including sacrificing our own lives. It unites us all.

It's a primitive response, a mixture of anger, longing and despair. It breaks through our sophistication. Often it does this in such small ways that we don't recognise it, brush it aside. When I separated myself from my babies after three months' maternity leave, taking my leaking breasts and podgy tummy back into the office, it felt strange. Yet I didn't let myself think too much about it, think that it was unnatural, cruel even, barbaric. Sometimes I told myself that it was my choice to leave my children, sometimes that I had no choice. Both were true. I enjoyed my work. We needed the money. But it was also true that most of my generation felt, quite rightly, that if they abandoned their hard-won careers, they would never pick them up again. So, like so many others, I rode roughly over my intense feelings of connection with my children, my natural impulses, and I made a kind of peace with myself, compromising as do millions of mothers every day. I found a good nanny and willingly gave up all my non-work time to my children. My cancer destroyed the notion that I could keep my children safe though and I was driven almost mad by the impossibility of my situation.

The problem, as I suddenly now saw it, was this: protecting my children, keeping them safe, no longer required that I do something, not that I even lay down my life for them, but that I do the opposite, that I not do something, that I not die. And that was not something I could wangle. It would or would not happen. And although I say that this was the problem I faced, it is not a problem that has gone away. Not a day goes by when I do not think about it. I am racked by guilt that it is beyond my ability to will myself to live for my children and that, however much they understand or can articulate what they feel about my health, the simple fact that I have been diagnosed with cancer has, in so many ways, ruined their lives. When I tell people this, they say one of two things. The first is: don't be ridiculous, it's not your fault. Of course it's not my fault. But fault is not the issue. The second is: don't be ridiculous, of course you haven't ruined their lives. This is wishful thinking, as is the notion that my illness has made my children better people, more empathic, rounded, that the changes it has triggered in their emotional make-up have been entirely benign.

I have, over the years, become acutely aware of what it means to be a motherless child in our society. I see things differently. Children's stories take on new poignancy – *Peter Pan*, *The Secret Garden*, *A Little Princess*. When I read interviews in magazines and newspapers, I am alert to the detail of the loss of a mother. It leaps out of the page at me. It might as well be highlighted in fluorescent pink. I am a republican and have never had any interest in the royal family – meeting the Princess of Wales was one of the less-interesting events of my life – but I still find myself pondering the future of the princes, William and Harry, as young men without a mother. Madonna, Bob

Geldof, Stella McCartney, Eddie Izzard. I look at them and wonder, how has that panned out? What do they remember about their mothers? How did they manage? And, of course, what did it feel like for their mothers knowing they were leaving them? I did know a mother who was dying and, in theory, I could have asked her this question, but I didn't. I couldn't bear to and, anyway, I knew what the answer would be. You do, too.

When it came to choosing a secondary school for Lucian, one of the most important considerations for me, next to academic standing, was that the school have a sense of community and good pastoral care. The quiet support from his primary school had been invaluable when I was ill and I wanted to be sure that it would be there again should anything happen to me. When he got into the school we all liked most, I felt as if I'd won the roll-over on the lottery – and sad that I needed to take such things so seriously.

There is, of course, no way I can ever know how my children will grow up if I die. There is also no way of knowing what effect my being ill has had on them. I cannot rewind the tape and watch them grow up without it. There is no possibility of a nice, neat blind trial. What I do know for sure though, and what I mean when I say I feel I have ruined their lives, is that I have failed in my duty as a mother to protect them from the monsters under the bed. I have introduced into their lives a sense of uncertainty. I am fallible. I have not always been there for them. This is something we all eventually learn about our parents as we grow up, but I am heartbroken that my children had to learn it at such a young age and in such a cruel way.

When I was diagnosed, Lucian was six and Cosima three.

Lucian was at school, Cosima at nursery. Kerry then looked after them until Simon or I got home from work. Throughout my treatment, in the most banal of ways, their lives did not change. It was not disrupted in that they did not miss school or nursery. Kerry still brought them home. They did not have to be looked after, as some children have to be in similar circumstances, by relatives, away from home. But I changed and that was a profound change.

I never hid my illness from them. I explained to them that I had breast cancer, that I had a lump in my right breast that had to be removed because it wasn't supposed to be there; the chemotherapy and radiotherapy was to stop it growing back again. I showed them the scars, the reconstruction. I never discussed the implications of my diagnosis with them. I thought about it. I didn't want to be feeble. I wanted to be strong for them. But there was nothing to say in the end. I didn't know what was going to happen to me and it seemed sadistic to tell them that there might be even bigger monsters lurking under the bed. I never lied. I simply stuck to the facts, an entirely inadequate description of my own experience, but a useful one for two small children. How much did they take in?

My experience of their distress or lack of it was patchy because my mothering was patchy during my treatment. I had always worked full-time, so the children were used to being away from me in the daytime. But I was always there when I wasn't working. I had no social life. I didn't want one. I wanted to be with them when I wasn't at work. When I became ill, this ability to dictate how I spent my time was almost entirely destroyed. I was hospitalised for the quadrantectomy, the mastectomy, the stem cell harvest, my first chemo session and the stem cell transplant itself. In between these brutal separations when I saw the children only occasionally, I was mainly at home, so then they saw more of me than they would have done normally. But I was often unwell, sometimes in bed, often lying on the sofa. I was fragile, I had little energy and I looked awful. I was not, in so many ways, the mother I had been. I frequently felt like a negative in their lives, a negative in that I had little positive to offer and a negative as in a photographic negative, faint, difficult to discern without close scrutiny.

The other important people in their lives — Simon, Kerry, my parents — valiantly substituted for me. Whenever I was hospitalised over a weekend, the children went to my parents. When I had the stem cell transplant, my mother took the children and Kerry to Disneyland Paris for a long weekend and Kerry took them to stay with her father in Cornwall for a while. Throughout my treatment, my mother and Kerry babysat whenever Simon needed to be with me at the hospital in the evening. I felt so lucky to have such support, but also so angry that I needed it.

Now when I ask the children what they can remember about me being ill, they don't seem to remember anything specific. They remember going to Disneyland, the hotel, the rides, the parades, but seem surprised when I tell them when they went. They remember a hospital bed, somewhere, they are not sure, that zoomed up and down. Cosima recently, after a storyline about breast cancer on *Neighbours*, asked me a torrent of questions about when I was ill. Did I have chemotherapy? Did I lose my hair, too? I told her I was surprised that she could not remember and she just shrugged her shoulders. But my instinct is that just because my children often cannot conjure up specifics for me that does not mean that they are untouched by the experience, that they have forgotten it. What do any of us remember specifically about certain periods of our childhoods? Holidays? Christmas presents? Falling off our bike? We all have our anecdotes but they are not the sum of our lives. We learn early the power of anecdotes. We learn that they oil the wheels of conversation. Vague ramblings about feelings, on the other hand, do not, but these feelings are what our lives are really about, what shape us until, in adult life, we are looking at something rather splendid, or its many-faceted opposite.

My children will have missed me when I was ill, been confused by my comings and goings, my inability to mother them as I had before, alarmed by the anxiety around them. Their ability to articulate these feelings would have been limited at the time, although not as limited as for many children of their age as they have always been encouraged to talk, explain themselves. Lucian, being older, obviously said more and often made me laugh with his astute analysis of my situation. Once, some time after my treatment had finished, I was lying on the sofa, reading a magazine, when he asked me to do something for him. I responded in a vague, not-now-Bernard way – it has to be said that one of the most frequently cited crimes I am accused of by my children is that I am 'always' lying on the sofa reading *The New Yorker* – but he was having none of it. 'You're not having your chemotherapy now, you know. Do it.' But however much the children were encouraged to talk, there were limits to their expressive powers and, in the same way that I was too wrapped up in the moment to understand my feelings, work through them, I suspect that they were, too.

What has happened since then, I believe, is that they, again like me, have slowly processed the feelings, the trauma they experienced then. I believe this process is inevitable but how it has manifested itself I have little idea. I have hunches – other people are wonderfully confident, informing me in ringing tones that the reason Lucian is such a way and Cosima that way is a direct result of my illness – but I find it impossible to be so sure. There is no way of knowing how they would have developed if I had not been ill. They do have a sensitivity to cancer that other children do not seem to have. When they hear about someone having cancer – from friends, or on the TV – they always ask what type it is. They also know that some people die from it and some people don't, but I can tell that the uncertainty about who will and who won't unsettles them. But I do feel that it is their prerogative to decide how they have been affected, not mine or anyone else's. My role is simple, to support them, to listen and to be alert to any connections to that dark time, however obscure, so that their feelings do not become distorted, diverted into unhelpful cul-de-sacs. It is also, of course, their prerogative to decide when they are older whether or not I have done this successfully.

I don't have a problem with children blaming parents for the way they were brought up. I agree with the poet Philip Larkin that our parents do fuck us up and I don't agree with the writer Martin Amis that the moment our children are born we forgive our parents everything. I'm not a masochist. I just think that our experience of our parents shapes us, full stop. As parents, we cannot pick and choose which bits of our personalities and lives tumble down the generations. We just have to find a way to deal with the consequences.

One of my worries is that my children have a highly developed sense of separation. It may be that I am hyper-alert to this tendency. It may be that it is me that has the problem to which they are responding. But my instinct is that a natural tendency has been exacerbated by my illness and that sometimes everyday separations are a subconscious reminder of those painful, earlier separations and therefore more upsetting than they would ordinarily be.

And what can I do about this? All I can do is support them, but at the back – and sometimes at the front – of my mind whenever I have to deal with any separation is my own complicated relationship with it. I am torn. Sometimes I feel I ought to spend every minute of the day with them, supporting them, because I do not know how long I have got with them. Other times, I feel I ought to put my energies into encouraging their independence because they may need to be more indepen- dent than most children, or at least independent of their mother. In my mind, I see-saw between these two oughts. They are just there. I cannot get them out of my mind and, boy, have I tried because what I long for more than anything else is to have a relationship with my children that is not so loaded, that is lighter. But the horrible thoughts creep up on me. They catch me unawares during the tiny moments and leave me undone.

It is a winter afternoon. We are at the cottage, sitting round the fire, listening to the afternoon play on the radio. I am making a tapestry with Cosima. Then suddenly I am overcome with despair. Who would do this with her if I died? I have to walk out of the room, do something, anything, to stop myself sobbing.

When I taught her how to knit and within hours I could watch her clacking away with confidence, I was thrilled, but I also thought how I might have missed this. I am so lucky I didn't.

Lucian needs some new clothes. We go shopping. We shop well together. We lark around, pondering the merits of this hoodie against that, try on 20 pairs of sunglasses before deciding which does the trick. We go to McDonald's, Lucian to eat, me to drink the disgusting coffee, and to mull over our excellent choices. And while we are chatting and laughing, a sick feeling sometimes rises up in me as I wonder who would have done this with him if I had not survived.

Their father would, of course. But it would not be the same. How could it be? A mother and a father are not interchangeable, and nor should they be. I don't mean that fathers are for playing football and mothers for washing football kits – after all, where would that leave our daughters – but they provide different role models, often hopeless, often downright odd, but role models nonetheless which give our children something to grapple with, copy or rebel against. It is confusing, unbalanced, when there is an absence.

Often the death of a mother in childhood – or at least before a new adult life has been created – triggers an idealisation of that mother. The abrupt separation interrupts a natural process of gradual separation. In fact, the disruption of the mother–child bond seems unnatural in every way I can imagine, and no matter how much some men say otherwise and whether or not it is nature or nurture, it seems worse than the disruption of the father–child bond. But maybe that is wrong, simply my own narcissism. Single-parent fathers are unusual. I have only met two children without mothers, both my son's age. The fathers and sons struggle to make a family life. But it is hard to unpick how much this is to do with the men themselves, their situation, seen as tragic, or because our attitudes towards mothers and fathers are so biased and entrenched. Most of the children I have met who live with their mothers – and there are many – because their parents are divorced or because their mothers chose to be single parents are infected by the idea that men are second-class parents. It's not necessarily because their mothers complain about them – although usually they do – but because the men are not the main event. They're not around, they're unreliable. They're not there for the tiny moments. It is baffling to me as to why so many men allow themselves to become such absences. But they do, even in two-parent families.

Many mothers I know have given up on their partners' ability to bond with their children, to engage with the detail of their children's lives, the intense disappointment they experienced during the baby years having given way to a weary resignation and sadness. They live with the fact that their partners don't know the name of their children's teachers, their shoe size, when half term falls, who their children's friends are. Woody Allen's semi-detached approach to fatherhood, as revealed in his court case with Mia Farrow, came as no surprise to most women – whether working or not – who get on with organising their children's lives while their partners dip in and out as it suits them.

There is a pay-off for women: becoming absolutely central to children's lives; and this power, in a world in which women still have relatively little power, is seductive. A dominant mother becomes the person her children adore most, hug first, call for in public. It's some compensation for the hard graft. But it leaves a bitter taste and leaves the unsatisfactory status quo unchanged.

For me, there can be no such compromise. A natural inclination to equality has become an intense desire. It is essential that my children have as meaningful and workable a relationship with Simon as they do with me, which is emotionally and practically enriching, and to enable that to flourish, I have to both do more and step back more than some mothers. It is something I have to do with deliberation, but it is not so hard. Simon is a wonderful father. He loves the children as much as I do. The children love him. He is also practical. He cooks, he shops, he drives, he gardens, he grows vegetables, makes jam, chutney. He is better than me at getting up in the night and getting up early. But he is a man. As I say, the sexes are not interchangeable. He doesn't naturally tune into the detail, the nail-cutting, the dental appointments, the homework timetable. He can organise all these things, but only if reminded. If I had never been ill, I am sure that like most of my friends, I would have let it go, but I'm too anxious to now. So I have consciously made the time to share the details with him. He has to know. Just in case.

Having Kerry in our lives protected me to a certain extent from these just-in-case fears. She had the detail in her head, too, and her presence meant that many aspects of parenthood were shared. Simon and I trusted her completely, and she was so warm and capable that she often felt like a third parent. Not surprisingly, when she left, when Simon and I both lost our jobs, I felt distressed. In one six-month period, I lost all financial security, I had to deal with the children's grief – I cannot describe it as anything else – at losing Kerry who had been part of their lives since they were born, and my own fears, so coloured by my cancer, about my responsibilities as a mother and my role as a mother. The ensuing months were hard as Simon and I struggled to take up the slack, to redistribute the workload of parenting and I was forced, very starkly, to face my own concerns about that detail.

This isn't fanciful. In Allison Pearson's novel *I Don't Know How She Does It*, her heroine Kate Reddy has a colleague whose wife dies of cancer. She was a full-time mother and she leaves her husband what sounds like a book of information about the detail of their family life. Most working mothers could write such a book, too. Simon and I are reading the book together though and, in doing so, I give up my place as the centre of my children's universe. It's a funny feeling. It fills me with both joy and sadness. Recently I sat in on a singing lesson with Cosima. They were working on a song from the musical *Oliver!* called 'Where is Love?'. Cosima was asked if she knew what the song was about. To prompt her, the teacher asked her who she was most pleased to see at the end of the day after school. Cosima got the hint and said that the song was about Oliver not having a mother. The teacher then asked her to imagine the feelings he had and reminded her how lovely it was to see mum at the school gates. Cosima looked at her calmly.

'Or dad,' she said. *I punched the air, without moving a muscle, of course.*

Over the years, I have had to get used to the fact that I am hard-wired like this, to my children's future. I used to weep whenever I glimpsed them from afar, laughing and playing together. For a long time, I found it hard to find pleasure in motherhood, so tainted had it become for me. But the exhilaration gradually came back. I can vividly remember the first time I tasted it. We were at the cottage sometime after my treatment was over. When the children were fractious, I would often put on music loudly and we would dance around the kitchen. It always worked, shaking off their bad mood. Abba was a winner, so much so that the children still think I genuinely like Abba and that 'Dancing Queen' is one of my favourite records. For many months I couldn't dance though. I felt immobilised with despair whenever I heard those jaunty lyrics. Then suddenly one wintry afternoon, I was up and whirling round the room, holding hands with Lucian, Cosima and Simon, and I was laughing. It was a breathtaking moment.

And now I mostly don't weep over my children. Or I do, but not as often. Sometimes I even fantasise about what it would be like to not have these worries, to assume, like most people, that things will be okay, but that feels dodgy. Mainly, I stick to the basics, trying to be a good mother, to give my children as much love as I can. On my printer, I have a quote from the psychotherapist Elaine Heffner, which says: 'The art of mothering is to teach the art of living to children.' That'll do. And I am so proud of my children. They are so beautiful and clever and charming. They often ask me what the best day of my life was and I always tell them, quite truthfully, that I have had two, the days they were born. And, of course, the worst day of my life was the day I was diagnosed with cancer, destroying my ordinary dreams of parenthood. I believe R. D. Laing when he says that we never truly know each other, but I know that I love what I see when I look at my children.

When my own father died, I wrote a tribute from 'the children'. It ended with this thought: 'Shortly before he died, our dad started to wonder what it meant to have a successful life. He didn't realise that he'd long ago given us children the answer to this question. By his example, he had taught us that, whatever happens in life, love is all you need.'

Everyone seemed to find it apt, but a couple of days after the funeral, I realised that I had been talking to myself about myself again. It was clear to me that the kindness of strangers, the doctors who had sorted out my malfunctioning body, Mrs Witham who had helped me sort out my troubled mind, would only ever be part of the story of my survival. These strangers had saved my life, my sanity. But they had saved me so that there might be more time with the other people in this story, the people who saved my life in a different way. My parents, my siblings, my friends, particularly Anna and Kerry. But most of all, Simon, Lucian and Cosima. The trinity of love. Maybe that's why I really fancied changing my name to Trinity.

Postscript

Less than a month after I finished this book, I discovered that the bad back I was suffering from was being caused by the return of my cancer. It had come back in my bones and also my liver. I had moved into a different waiting room, this one nearer the exit. I was devastated. But, after the initial shock subsided, I began to realise that I was not in such a different place. There was cautious, albeit more cautious than ever before, optimism from my doctors and I was facing an unknown future, much as I had been for the last seven years, which demanded a certain stoicism and a positive attitude of me – not a daft, Pollyanna-style attitude but a willingness to throw myself into my treatment – and life – with enthusiasm. As I write, my treatment has consisted of radiotherapy and the beginning of a course of chemotherapy. As I write, I am also still a cancer survivor and my priorities remain unchanged. Through the din of all the other anxieties clamouring for my attention, one can be heard louder and clearer: how to seize the day with Simon and Lucian and Cosima. The road ahead looks forbidding, but I won't be put off. I can't afford to be. There's too much at stake, both for myself and my precious family.

Bibliography

Clarke, Jane *Body Foods for Women*, Orion, London, 1997.

Didion, Joan *The White Album*, Flamingo, 1993.

Lorde, Audre *Cancer Journals*, Spinsters Ink, US, 1982.

Love, Susan *Dr Susan Love's Breast Book*, Perseus Publishing, 2000.

Moore, Oscar *PWA: Looking AIDS in the Face*, Picador, London, 1996.

Phillips, Adam *Darwin's Worms*, Faber and Faber, London, 1999.

Phillips, Adam *On Kissing, Tickling and Being Bored: Psychoanalytic Essays on the Unexamined Life*, Faber and Faber, London, 1994.

Phillips, Adam *Promises, Promises: Essays on Literature and Psychoanalysis*, Faber and Faber, London, 2002.

Phillips, Adam *Terrors and Experts*, Faber and Faber, London, 1997.

Rinpoche, Sogyal *The Tibetan Book of Living and Dying*, Rider, London, 2002.

Sontag, Susan *Illness as Metaphor*, Penguin Books, London, 2002.

Stoppard, Miriam *The Breast Book*, Dk Pub, London, 1996

White, Edmund *Farewell Symphony*, Chatto and Windus, London, 1997.

Woolf, Virginia *On Being Ill*, Consortium, 2002.

How To Help Yourself

BACP – The British Association for Counselling and Psychotherapy
BACP House
35–37 Albert Street
Rugby
Warwickshire
CV21 2SG
Tel: 0870 443 5252
Email: bacp@bacp.co.uk
Website: www.bacp.co.uk

Breast Cancer Care
Kiln House
210 New Kings Road
London
SW6 4NZ
Helpline: 0808 800 6000
Tel: 020 7384 2984
Fax: 020 7384 3387
Email: info@breastcancercare.org.uk
Website: www.breastcancercare.org.uk

CancerBACUP
3 Bath Place
Rivington Street
London
EC2A 3JR
Helpline: 0808 800 1234
Tel: 020 7696 9003
Fax: 020 7696 9002
Website: www.cancerbacup.org.uk

The Cancer Counselling Trust
1 Noel Road
London
N1 8HQ
Tel: 020 7704 1137
Fax: 020 7704 8620
Email: support@cctrust.org.uk
Website: www.cctrust.org.uk

Julie Friedeberger
Since Julie's experience of breast cancer in 1993, her focus has been on yoga as a healing therapy, and on the power of simple movements, breathing and relaxation to help in the healing process. Julie is contactable through The Yoga Biomedical Trust: www.yogatherapy.org

Gilda's Club Worldwide
322 Eighth Avenue
Suite 1402
New York
NY 10001
USA
Email: info@gildasclub.org
Website: www.gildasclub.org

Ruby Lawson
Yoga teacher: individuals and groups.
Tel: 020 7352 5925

Maggie's Centre
Maggie's Edinburgh
The Stables
Western General Hospital
Crewe Road South
Edinburgh
EH4 2XU
Tel: 0131 537 3131
Fax: 0131 537 3130
Email: maggies.centre@ed.ac.uk
Website: www.maggiescentres.org

Index

C
Because cowards get cancer too
John Diamond

'…a fearlessly honest account that has already been hailed as a modern classic' *The Guardian*

Part journal, part medical enquiry, this bestselling book is the everyday story of cancer: what it is, what it does, how it kills and how it can be cured.

Consciously Female
A groundbreaking programme to help you feel great every day of the month, every month of your life
Tracy Gaudet

Dr Gaudet shows women how to reframe what it means to live inside a woman's body – so instead of crossing off the days we feel bad, we learn to understand them as part of an important cycle in our lives. Her complete wellness programme combines conventional and alternative medicine with advice on nutrition, exercise, rituals and mind-body techniques. It is positive, practical and inspirational – and it's for every woman.

Dr Ali's Nutrition Bible
Dramatically improve the way you feel with this pioneering approach to eating from the UK's leading integrated health specialist
Dr Mosaraf Ali

The definitive nutrition bible for the 21st century, this pioneering book allows you to choose the best way of eating to suit your individual situation. Based on age, gender, temperament, lifestyle and state of health, the book provides an easy-to-follow companion to healthy eating, with information on all the nutritional basics for a balanced diet. There is also an extensive section on dietary solutions to health problems, including diabetes, colds and flu, IBS, arthritis, high blood pressure, anxiety and eczema.

☐ **C**	0091816653	£7.99
☐ **Consciously Female**	009188229X	£12.99
☐ **Dr Ali's Nutrition Bible**	0091889499	£20.00

FREE POST AND PACKING

Overseas customers allow £2.00 per paperback

BY PHONE: 01624 677237

BY POST: Random House Books
c/o Bookpost
PO Box 29
Douglas
Isle of Man, IM99 1BQ

BY FAX: 01624 670923

BY EMAIL: bookshop@enterprise.net

Cheques (payable to Bookpost) and credit cards accepted

Prices and availability subject to change without notice.
Allow 28 days for delivery.
When placing your order, please mention if you do not wish to receive
any additional information

www.randomhouse.co.uk